MILITARY AND VETERAN ISSUES

MILITARY MEDICAL CARE AND VETERANS HEALTH CARE

QUESTIONS AND ANSWERS

MILITARY AND VETERAN ISSUES

Additional books in this series can be found on Nova's website under the Series tab.

Additional e-books in this series can be found on Nova's website under the e-book tab.

MILITARY AND VETERAN ISSUES

MILITARY MEDICAL CARE AND VETERANS HEALTH CARE

QUESTIONS AND ANSWERS

ADAM SEWARD
EDITOR

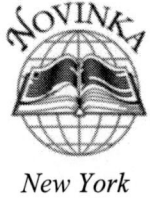

New York

Copyright © 2014 by Nova Science Publishers, Inc.

All rights reserved. No part of this book may be reproduced, stored in a retrieval system or transmitted in any form or by any means: electronic, electrostatic, magnetic, tape, mechanical photocopying, recording or otherwise without the written permission of the Publisher.

For permission to use material from this book please contact us:
Telephone 631-231-7269; Fax 631-231-8175
Web Site: http://www.novapublishers.com

NOTICE TO THE READER

The Publisher has taken reasonable care in the preparation of this book, but makes no expressed or implied warranty of any kind and assumes no responsibility for any errors or omissions. No liability is assumed for incidental or consequential damages in connection with or arising out of information contained in this book. The Publisher shall not be liable for any special, consequential, or exemplary damages resulting, in whole or in part, from the readers' use of, or reliance upon, this material. Any parts of this book based on government reports are so indicated and copyright is claimed for those parts to the extent applicable to compilations of such works.

Independent verification should be sought for any data, advice or recommendations contained in this book. In addition, no responsibility is assumed by the publisher for any injury and/or damage to persons or property arising from any methods, products, instructions, ideas or otherwise contained in this publication.

This publication is designed to provide accurate and authoritative information with regard to the subject matter covered herein. It is sold with the clear understanding that the Publisher is not engaged in rendering legal or any other professional services. If legal or any other expert assistance is required, the services of a competent person should be sought. FROM A DECLARATION OF PARTICIPANTS JOINTLY ADOPTED BY A COMMITTEE OF THE AMERICAN BAR ASSOCIATION AND A COMMITTEE OF PUBLISHERS.

Additional color graphics may be available in the e-book version of this book.

Library of Congress Cataloging-in-Publication Data

ISBN: 978-1-63117-531-2

Published by Nova Science Publishers, Inc. † New York

CONTENTS

Preface		vii
Chapter 1	Military Medical Care: Questions and Answers *Don J. Jansen*	1
Chapter 2	Health Care for Veterans: Answers to Frequently Asked Questions *Sidath Viranga Panangala and Erin Bagalman*	35
Index		65

PREFACE

This book answers several frequently asked questions about military health care, and provides responses to frequently asked questions about health care provided to veterans through the Veterans Health Administration.

Chapter 1 – The primary objective of the military health system, which includes the Defense Department's hospitals, clinics, and medical personnel, is to maintain the health of military personnel so they can carry out their military missions and to be prepared to deliver health care during wartime. The military health system also covers dependents of active duty personnel, military retirees, and their dependents, including some members of the reserve components. The military health system provides health care services through either Department of Defense (DOD) medical facilities, known as "military treatment facilities" or "MTFs" as space is available, or through private health care providers. The military health system serves 9.7 million beneficiaries through care purchased from private providers as well as directly through a system of DOD military treatment facilities that currently includes some 56 hospitals and 365 clinics. It operates worldwide and employs some 58,369 civilians and 86,007 military personnel.

Since 1966, civilian care to millions of dependents and retirees (and retirees' dependents) has been provided through a program still known in law as the Civilian Health and Medical Program of the Uniformed Services (CHAMPUS), but more commonly known as TRICARE. TRICARE has four main benefit plans: a health maintenance organization option (TRICARE Prime), a preferred provider option (TRICARE Extra), a fee-for-service option (TRICARE Standard), and a Medicare wrap-around option (TRICARE for Life) for Medicare-eligible retirees. Other TRICARE plans include TRICARE Young Adult, TRICARE Reserve Select and TRICARE Retired Reserve.

TRICARE also includes a pharmacy program and optional dental plans. Options available to beneficiaries vary by the beneficiary's duty status and location.

This report answers several frequently asked questions about military health care, including

- How is the military health system structured?
- What is TRICARE?
- What are the different TRICARE plans and who is eligible?
- What are the costs of military health care to beneficiaries?
- What is the relationship of TRICARE to Medicare?
- How does the Affordable Care Act affect TRICARE?
- What are the long-term trends in defense health care costs?
- What is the Medicare Eligible Retiree Health Care fund, which funds TRICARE for Life?

This report does not address issues specific to battlefield medicine, veterans, or the Veterans Health Administration.

Chapter 2 – The Veterans Health Administration (VHA), within the Department of Veterans Affairs (VA), operates the nation's largest integrated health care delivery system, provides care to more than 5.5 million veteran patients, and employs more than 258,000 full-time equivalent employees.

Eligibility and Enrollment. Contrary to claims concerning promises of "free health care for life," not every veteran is automatically entitled to medical care from the VA. Eligibility for VA health care is based primarily on veteran status resulting from military service. Generally, veterans must also meet minimum service requirements; however, exceptions are made for veterans discharged due to service-connected disabilities, members of the Reserve and National Guard (under certain circumstances), and returning combat veterans. The VA categorizes veterans into eight Priority Groups, based on factors such as service-connected disabilities and income (among others). Dependents, caregivers, and survivors of certain veterans are eligible for the Civilian Health and Medical Program of the Department of Veterans Affairs (CHAMPVA), which reimburses non-VA providers or facilities for their medical care.

Medical Benefits. All enrolled veterans are offered a standard medical benefits package, which includes (but is not limited to) inpatient and outpatient medical services, pharmaceuticals, durable medical equipment, and prosthetic devices.

For female veterans, the VA provides gender-specific care, such as gynecological care, breast and reproductive oncology, infertility treatment, maternity care, and care for conditions related to military sexual trauma. Under current regulations, the VA is not authorized to provide, or cover the costs of, in vitro fertilization, abortion counseling, abortions, or medication to induce abortions.

Generally the VA provides audiology and eye care services (including preventive services and routine vision testing) for all enrolled veterans, but eyeglasses and hearing aids are provided only to veterans meeting certain criteria. Eligibility for VA dental care is limited and differs significantly from eligibility for medical care. For veterans with service-connected disabilities who meet certain criteria, the VA provides short- and long-term nursing care, respite, and end-oflife care.

Under certain circumstances, the VA may reimburse non-VA providers for health care services rendered to VA-enrolled veterans on a fee-for-service basis. Such Fee Basis Care may include outpatient care, inpatient care, emergency care, medical transportation, and dental services.

Costs to Veterans and Insurance Collections. While enrolled veterans do not pay premiums for VA care, some veterans are required to pay copayments for medical services and outpatient medications related to the treatment of nonservice-connected conditions. Copayment amounts vary by Priority Group and type of service (e.g., inpatient versus outpatient). The VA has the authority to bill most health care insurers for nonservice-connected care; any insurer's payment received by the VA is used to offset "dollar for dollar" a veteran's VA copayment responsibility. The VA is statutorily prohibited from receiving Medicare payments (with a narrow exception).

In: Military Medical Care ...
Editor: Adam Seward

ISBN: 978-1-63117-531-2
© 2014 Nova Science Publishers, Inc.

Chapter 1

MILITARY MEDICAL CARE: QUESTIONS AND ANSWERS[*]

Don J. Jansen

SUMMARY

The primary objective of the military health system, which includes the Defense Department's hospitals, clinics, and medical personnel, is to maintain the health of military personnel so they can carry out their military missions and to be prepared to deliver health care during wartime. The military health system also covers dependents of active duty personnel, military retirees, and their dependents, including some members of the reserve components. The military health system provides health care services through either Department of Defense (DOD) medical facilities, known as "military treatment facilities" or "MTFs" as space is available, or through private health care providers. The military health system serves 9.7 million beneficiaries through care purchased from private providers as well as directly through a system of DOD military treatment facilities that currently includes some 56 hospitals and 365 clinics. It operates worldwide and employs some 58,369 civilians and 86,007 military personnel.

Since 1966, civilian care to millions of dependents and retirees (and retirees' dependents) has been provided through a program still known in

---

[*] This is an edited, reformatted and augmented version of a Congressional Research Service publication, CRS Report for Congress RL33537, from www.crs.gov, prepared for Members and Committees of Congress, dated January 2, 2014.

law as the Civilian Health and Medical Program of the Uniformed Services (CHAMPUS), but more commonly known as TRICARE. TRICARE has four main benefit plans: a health maintenance organization option (TRICARE Prime), a preferred provider option (TRICARE Extra), a fee-for-service option (TRICARE Standard), and a Medicare wrap-around option (TRICARE for Life) for Medicare-eligible retirees. Other TRICARE plans include TRICARE Young Adult, TRICARE Reserve Select and TRICARE Retired Reserve. TRICARE also includes a pharmacy program and optional dental plans. Options available to beneficiaries vary by the beneficiary's duty status and location.

This report answers several frequently asked questions about military health care, including

- How is the military health system structured?
- What is TRICARE?
- What are the different TRICARE plans and who is eligible?
- What are the costs of military health care to beneficiaries?
- What is the relationship of TRICARE to Medicare?
- How does the Affordable Care Act affect TRICARE?
- What are the long-term trends in defense health care costs?
- What is the Medicare Eligible Retiree Health Care fund, which funds TRICARE for Life?

This report does not address issues specific to battlefield medicine, veterans, or the Veterans Health Administration.

BACKGROUND

Since 1966, civilian healthcare to millions of service members' dependents and retirees (and retirees' dependents) has been provided through a program still known in law as the Civilian Health and Medical Program of the Uniformed Services (CHAMPUS), but more commonly known as TRICARE. The "TRI" in "TRICARE" originally referred to the three main main benefit plan options: a health maintenance organization option (TRICARE Prime), a preferred provider option (TRICARE Extra), and a fee-for-service option (TRICARE Standard). A Medicare wrap-around option (TRICARE for Life) for Medicare-eligible retirees was added in 2002. Other TRICARE plans include TRICARE Young Adult, TRICARE Reserve Select, and TRICARE Retired Reserve. TRICARE also includes a pharmacy program and optional dental plans. Options available to beneficiaries vary by the beneficiary's duty status and location.

The Government Accountability Office (GAO) and the Congressional Budget Office (CBO) have also published important studies on the organization, coordination, and costs of the military health system, as well as its effectiveness addressing particular health challenges. Another source of information is the Office of the Assistant Secretary of Defense for Health Affairs Home Page.[1]

QUESTIONS AND ANSWERS

1. How Is the Military Health System Structured?

The Military Health System (MHS) restructured in the fall of 2013 and is now primarily administered by a new entity known as the Defense Health Agency (DHA). As described in the most recent DOD report to Congress on MHS administration, this resulted in the several new leadership organizations described below.[2] In addition, during 2013 a new round of regional managed care support contracts fully took effect.

Leadership

The Military Health System Executive Review (MHSER) serves as a senior-level forum for DOD leadership input into the strategic, transitional, and emerging issues. The MHSER advises the Office of the Secretary of Defense (SECDEF) and the Office of the Deputy Secretary of Defense (DEPSECDEF) about performance challenges and direction. The MHSER is chaired by the Under Secretary of Defense (Personnel and Readiness) (USD[P&R]), and includes the Principal Deputy Under Secretary of Defense (Personnel and Readiness), the Assistant Secretary of Defense (Health Affairs) (ASD[HA]), the service vice chiefs, military department assistant secretaries for manpower and reserve affairs, the Assistant Commandant of the Marine Corps, the Director of Program Analysis and Evaluation, the Principal Deputy Under Secretary of Defense (Comptroller), the Director of the Joint Staff, and the surgeons general (as ex-officio members).

The Senior Military Medical Action Council (SMMAC) is the highest governing body in the MHS. The SMMAC is chaired by the ASD(HA), and includes the Principal Deputy Assistant Secretary of Defense (Health Affairs) (PDASD[HA]), military department Surgeons General, DHA Director, Joint Staff Surgeon, and other attendees as required. The SMMAC presents enterprise-level guidance and operational issues for decision-making by the ASD(HA).

Reporting to the SMMAC is the Medical Deputies Action Group (MDAG), which ensures that actions are coordinated across the MHS and are in alignment with strategy, policies, directives, and initiatives of the MHS. The MDAG is chaired by the PDASD(HA), and includes the Deputy Surgeons General, DHA Deputy Director, and a Joint Staff Surgeon Representative.

Reporting to the MDAG are four supporting governing bodies:

- The Medical Operations Group (MOG) consists of the senior healthcare operations directors of the Service medical departments, the DHA Director of Healthcare Operations, and a Joint Staff Surgeon representative, with the chairmanship rotating among these members. The MOG carries out MDAG assigned tasks and provides a collaborative and transparent forum supporting enterprise-wide oversight of direct and purchased care systems focused on sustaining and improving the MHS.
- The Medical Business Operations Group (MBOG) consists of the senior resource managers of the Service medical departments and the DHA Director of Business Operations, with the chairmanship rotating among these members. The MBOG provides a forum for providing resource management input to the MDAG on direct and purchased care issues and initiatives focused on sustaining and improving the MHS.
- The Human Resources and Manpower Workgroup (HR&MAN POWER WG) consists of the senior human resources and manpower representatives from the Service medical departments and the DHA, with the chairmanship rotating among these members. The HR&MANPOWER WG supports centralized, coordinated policy execution, and guidance for development of coordinated human resources and manpower policies and procedures for the MHS.
- The Enhanced Multi-Service Markets (eMSM) Leadership Group. eMSMs are geographic MHS markets served by more than one military department under the direction of a designated Market Manager with enhanced authorities. The six eMSMs are:
1) Tidewater, Virginia
2) Puget Sound, Washington
3) Colorado Springs, Colorado
4) San Antonio, Texas

5) Oahu, Hawaii
6) National Capital Region
- The eMSM Leadership Group is composed of the sixMarket Managers, with the chairmanship rotating among these members. The eMSM Leadership Group

Finally, the ASD(HA) is supported and advised by the Policy Advisory Council (PAC), composed of the Deputy Assistant Secretaries of Defense (Health Affairs), the DHA Deputy Director, the Deputy Surgeons General, and a representative of the Joint Staff. The PAC provides a forum for supporting MHS-wide policy development and oversight in a unified manner.

Defense Health Agency

On the operational side, the Defense Health Agency (DHA) is designated as a Combat Support Agency in order to ensure that the DHA remains focused on the primary mission of medical readiness, and is responsive to the Combatant Commanders through a formal oversight process established by the Chairman, Joint Chiefs of Staff. The Assistant Secretary of Defense for Health Affairs (ASD(HA)) will provide the Deputy Secretary of Defense with a detailed plan for implementing a shared services model within the military health system. A "shared services model" means that the DHA will assume responsibility for shared services, functions, and activities in the military health system, including the TRICARE program, pharmacy programs, medical education and training, medical research and development, health information technology, facility planning, public health, medical logistics, acquisition, budget, and resource management. The current Joint Task Force National Capital Region Medical (JTF CAPMED) will be assigned to an organization subordinate to the DHA that will be known as the National Capital Region.

The military health system serving 9.7 million beneficiaries through care purchased from private providers as well as directly through a system of DOD military treatment facilities that currently includes some 56 hospitals and 365 clinics. It operates worldwide and employs approximately 68,000 civilians and 86,000 military personnel. Direct care costs include the provision of medical care directly to beneficiaries, the administrative requirements of a large medical establishment, and maintaining a capability to provide medical care to combat forces in case of hostilities. Civilian providers under contract to DOD have constituted a major portion of the defense health reconstruction in recent years.

TRICARE Regional Managed Health Care Support Contracts

TRICARE is administered through managed care support contracts in three regions:

- TRICARE North Region covering Connecticut, Delaware, the District of Columbia, Illinois, Indiana, Kentucky, Maine, Maryland, Massachusetts, Michigan, New Hampshire, New Jersey, New York, North Carolina, Ohio, Pennsylvania, Rhode Island, Vermont, Virginia, West Virginia, Wisconsin, and portions of Iowa, Missouri, and Tennessee. The TRICARE North regional contractor is currently Health Net Federal Services.
- TRICARE South Region covering Alabama, Arkansas, Florida, Georgia, Louisiana, Mississippi, Oklahoma, South Carolina, and most of Tennessee and Texas. The TRICARE South regional contractor is currently Humana Military Health Services.
- TRICARE West Region covering Alaska, Arizona, California, Colorado, Hawaii, Idaho, most of Iowa, Kansas, Minnesota, most of Missouri, Montana, Nebraska, Nevada, New Mexico, North Dakota, Oregon, South Dakota, portions of Texas, Utah, Washington, and Wyoming. The TRICARE West regional contractor is currently UnitedHealthcare.

These three contracts were re-competed in 2009, and after resolving bid protests, the new contracts known as "TRICARE Third Generation (T-3) Support Contracts" became operational between 2011 and 2012. Health care delivery under the new T-3 Contracts began April 1, 2011, for the North region with Health Net Federal Services. Humana Military Healthcare Services began health care delivery for TRICARE South region April 1, 2012. UnitedHealthcare began delivery of services to the TRICARE West region April 1, 2013.

2. What Is the Unified Medical Budget?

ASD(HA) prepares and submits a unified medical budget, which includes resources for the medical activities under his or her control within the DOD. The unified medical budget includes funding for all fixed medical treatment facilities/activities, including such costs as real property maintenance, environmental compliance, minor construction, and base operations support.

Funds for medical personnel and accrual payments to the Medicare Eligible Retiree Health Care Fund ((MERHCF)—see question "3. What is the Medicare Eligible Retiree Health Care Fund (MERHCF)?") are also included. The unified medical budget does not include resources associated with combat support medical units/activities. In these instances the funding responsibility is assigned to military service combatant or support commands.

Unified medical budget funding has traditionally been appropriated in several sources:

- The defense appropriations bill provides Operation and Maintenance (O&M), Procurement, and Research, Development, Test and Evaluation (RDT&E) funding under the heading "Defense Health Program."
- Funding for military medical personnel (doctors, corpsmen, and other health care providers) and TRICARE for Life accrual payments are generally provided in the defense appropriations bill under the "Military Personnel" (MILPERS) title.
- Funding for medical military construction (MILCON) is generally provided under the "Department of Defense" title of the military construction and veterans affairs bill.
- A standing authorization for transfers from the MERHCF to reimburse TRICARE for the cost of services provided to Medicare eligible retirees is provided by Section 1113 of title 10, United States Code (10 U.S.C. 1113).
- Costs of war-related military health care are generally funded through supplemental appropriations bills.

Other resources are made available to the military health system from third-party collections authorized by 10 U.S.C.1097b (b) and a number of other reimbursable program and transfer authorities. The President's budget typically refers to the unified medical budget request as its funding request for the military health system but only includes an exhibit for the DHP in the "Department of Defense—Military" chapter and exhibits for the MERHCF in the "Other Defense—Civil Programs" chapter of the Appendix volume. Medical MILCON and MILPERS request levels are generally found in DOD's budget submissions to Congress.

As illustrated in *Figure 1* below, the Obama Administration's FY2014 unified medical budget request[3] totals $49.4 billion and includes the following:

- $33.1 billion for the Defense Health Program (not including "Wounded, Ill, and Injured" funding);
- $8.5 billion for military personnel;
- $1.1 billion for medical military construction; and
- $6.7 billion for accrual payments to the MERHCF.

Much more detailed breakouts are available in budget exhibits published by the Department of Defense at http://www.budget.mil.

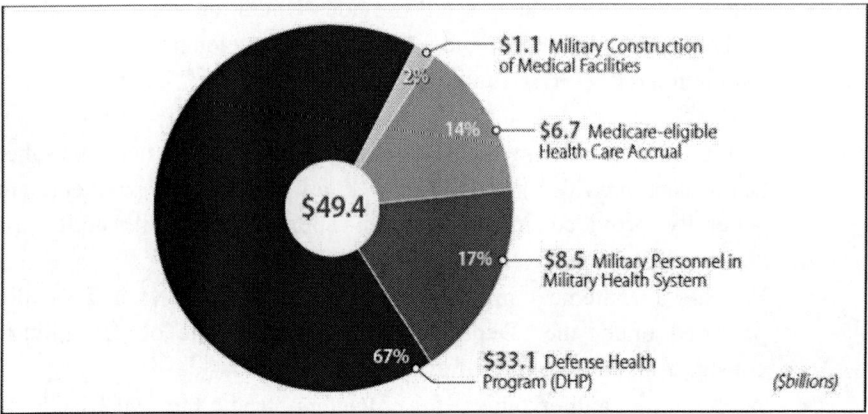

Source: Department of Defense FY2014 Budget Request Overview. Adapted by CRS Graphics.

Figure 1. FY2014 Unified Medical Budget Request ($billions).

3. What Is the Medicare Eligible Retiree Health Care Fund (MERHCF)?

The Floyd D. Spence National Defense Authorization Act for FY2001(FY2001 NDAA),[4] directed the establishment of the Medicare-Eligible Retiree Health Care Fund to pay for Medicare-eligible retiree health care beginning on October 1, 2002, via a new program called TRICARE for Life. Prior to this date, care for Medicare-eligible beneficiaries was space-available care in Military Treatment Facilities (MTF). The MERHCF covers Medicare-eligible beneficiaries, regardless of age.

The FY2001 NDAA also established an independent three-member DOD Medicare-Eligible Retiree Health Care Board of Actuaries appointed by the Secretary of Defense. Accrual deposits into the Fund are made by the agencies who employ future beneficiaries (DOD and the other uniformed services including the Public Health Service, the Coast Guard, and the National Oceanic & Atmospheric Administration) based upon estimates of future TRICARE for Life expenses. Transfers out are made to the Defense Health Program based on estimates of the cost of care actually provided each year. As of September 30, 2011, the Fund had assets of over $163.6 billion to cover future expenses.[5]

The Board is required to review the actuarial status of the fund, to report annually to the Secretary of Defense, and to report to the President and Congress on the status of the fund at least every four years. The DOD Office of the Actuary provides all technical and administrative support to the Board. Within DOD, the Office of the Under Secretary of Defense for Personnel and Readiness, through the Office of the Assistant Secretary of Defense (OASD) for Health Affairs (HA), has as one of its missions operational oversight of the defense health program including management of the MERHCF. The Defense Finance and Accounting Service provides accounting and investment services for the Fund.

4. What Is TRICARE?

The Dependents Medical Care Act of 1956[6] provided a statutory basis for dependents of active duty members, retirees, and dependents of retirees to seek care at MTFs. Prior to this time, authority for such care was fragmented. The 1956 act allowed DOD to contract for a health insurance plan for coverage of civilian hospital services for active duty dependents. Due to growing use of MTFs by eligible civilians and resource constraints, Congress adopted the Military Medical Benefits Amendments in 1966,[7] which allowed DOD to contract with civilian health providers to provide non-hospital-based care to eligible dependents and retirees. Since 1966, civilian care to millions of dependents and retirees (and retirees' dependents) has been provided through a program still known in law as the Civilian Health and Medical Program of the Uniformed Services (CHAMPUS), but since 1994 more commonly known as TRICARE.

TRICARE has four main benefit plans: a health maintenance organization option (TRICARE Prime), a preferred provider option (TRICARE Extra), a fee-for-service option (TRICARE Standard), and a Medicare wrap-around option (TRICARE for Life) for Medicare-eligible retirees. Other TRICARE plans include TRICARE Young Adult, TRICARE Reserve Select, and

TRICARE Retired Reserve. These plans are described below. TRICARE also includes a Pharmacy program and optional dental plans. Options available to beneficiaries vary by the beneficiary's relationship to a sponsor, sponsor's duty status, and location.

5. Who Is Eligible to Receive Care?

Eligibility for TRICARE is determined by the uniformed services and reported to the Defense Enrollment Eligibility Reporting System (DEERS). All eligible beneficiaries must have their eligibility status recorded in DEERS.

TRICARE beneficiaries can be divided into two main categories: sponsors and dependents. Sponsors are usually active duty servicemembers, National Guard/Reserve members, or retired servicemembers. "Sponsor" refers to the person who is serving or who has served on active duty or in the National Guard or Reserves. "Dependent" is defined in 10 U.S.C. 1072 and includes a variety of relationships, for example, spouses (including same-sex spouses), children, and certain unremarried former spouses.

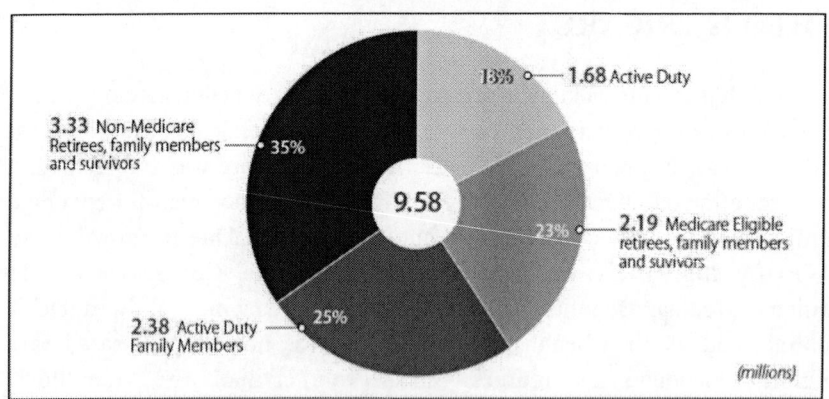

Source: The President's Budget for FY2013, Appendix, "Department of Defense–Military Programs," p. 271. Adapted by CRS.

Figure 2. Military Health System Eligible Beneficiaries. (millions).

6. What Are the Different TRICARE Plans? TRICARE Prime

TRICARE Prime is a managed healthcare option similar to a health maintenance organization. Like such civilian arrangements, the plan's features include a primary healthcare provider (either a military or a civilian health care provider) who manages care and provides or facilitates referrals to specialists. Referrals generally are required for such visits. To participate, beneficiaries must enroll and pay an annual enrollment fee, which is similar to an annual premium. Eligible beneficiaries may choose to enroll at any time. Enrollees receive first priority for appointments at military health care facilities and pay less out of pocket than do beneficiaries who use the other TRICARE plans. TRICARE Prime does not have an annual deductible.

Active duty servicemembers are required to use TRICARE Prime. Both they and their family members, as well as surviving spouses (during the first three years) and surviving dependent children, are exempt from the annual enrollment fee. Retired servicemembers, their families, surviving spouses (after the first three years), eligible former spouses, and others are required to pay an annual enrollment fee, which is applied to the annual catastrophic out-of-pocket-limit. TRICARE Prime annual enrollment fees for military retirees were increased in FY2012 for new enrollees for the first time since the program began. Moving forward, under 10 U.S.C. 1097(e) TRICARE Prime enrollment fees will be subject to increases each fiscal year based on the annual retirement pay cost-of-living adjustment for the calendar year. For FY2013 (October 1, 2012– September 30, 2013) this enrollment fee is $269.28 for an individual and $538.56 for individual plus family coverage.

TRICARE Standard

TRICARE Standard is a traditional fee-for-service (FFS) option that does not require beneficiaries to enroll in order to participate. TRICARE Standard plan allows participants to use authorized out-of-network civilian providers, but it also requires users to pay higher out-of-pocket costs, generally 25% of the allowable charge for retirees and 20% for active duty family members. TRICARE Standard requires an annual deductible of $150/individual or $300/family for family members of sponsors at pay grades E-5 and above and $50/$100 for pay grades E-4 and below. Beneficiaries who use the Standard option must pay any difference between a provider's billed charges and the rate of reimbursement allowed under the plan.

TRICARE Extra

TRICARE Extra is also available to TRICARE Standard beneficiaries. It also has no formal enrollment requirement and mirrors a civilian preferred provider network. Network providers agree to accept a reduced payment from TRICARE and to file all claims for participants. By using network providers under TRICARE Extra, beneficiaries reduce their copayments, in general, to 20% of the allowable charge for retirees and 15% for active duty family members.

TRICARE Reserve Select

The TRICARE Reserve Select program was authorized by Section 701 of the Ronald W. Reagan National Defense Authorization Act for FY2005 (P.L. 108-375), which enacted 10 U.S.C. 1076d. TRICARE Reserve Select is a premium-based health plan available worldwide for qualified Selected Reserve members of the Ready Reserve and their families. Servicemembers are not eligible for TRICARE Reserve Select if they are on active duty orders, covered under the Transitional Assistance Management Program, or eligible for or enrolled in the Federal Employees Health Benefits Program (FEHBP) or currently covered under the FEHBP through a family member. TRICARE Reserve Select provides benefits similar to TRICARE Standard. The government subsidizes the cost of the program with members paying 28% of the cost of the program in the form of premiums. For calendar year 2013, premiums were $51.62 per month for member only coverage, and $195.81 per month for member and family coverage. For calendar year 2014, TRICARE Reserve Select premiums are $51.68 per month for member only coverage, and $204.29 per month for member and family coverage.

TRICARE Retired Reserve

Section 705 of the National Defense Authorization Act for FY2010 (P.L. 111-84) added a new 10 U.S.C. 1076e to authorize a TRICARE coverage option for so-called "gray area" reservists, those who have retired but are too young to draw retirement pay. The program established under this authority is known as TRICARE Retired Reserve. Previously, such individuals were not eligible for any TRICARE coverage. This is a premium-based health plan that qualified retired members of the National Guard and Reserve under the age of 60 may purchase for themselves and eligible family members. It is similar to TRICARE Reserve Select, but differs in that there is no government subsidy as there is with TRICARE Reserve Select. As such, retired Reserve Component members who elect to purchase TRICARE Retired Reserve must pay the full cost of the calculated premium plus an additional administrative fee. Retired Reserve Component personnel who elect to participate in TRICARE Retired Reserve become eligible for the same TRICARE Standard,

TRICARE Extra, or TRICARE Prime options as active component retirees when the servicemember reaches age 60. Calendar year 2013 premiums for member only coverage were $402.11 per month and $969.10 per month for member-and-family plans. For calendar year 2014, TRICARE Retired Reserve premiums are $390.99 per month for member only coverage, and $956.65 per month for member and family coverage.

TRICARE Young Adult

Section 702 of the Ike Skelton National Defense Authorization Act for Fiscal Year 2011 (P.L. 111-383) added a new 10 U.S.C. 1110b, allowing unmarried children up to age 26, who are not otherwise eligible to enroll in an employer-sponsored plan, to purchase TRICARE coverage. The option established under this authority is known as "The TRICARE Young Adult Program." Unlike insurance coverage mandated by the Patient Protection and Affordable Care Act (P.L. 111-148), the TRICARE Young Adult Program provides individual coverage, rather than coverage under a family plan. A separate premium is charged. The law requires payment of a premium equal to the cost of the coverage as determined by the Secretary of Defense on an appropriate actuarial basis. For calendar year 2013 the monthly premium for a TRICARE Young Adult (TYA) Prime enrollment was $176 and $152 for a TYA Standard enrollment. For calendar year 2013 the monthly premium for a TRICARE Young Adult (TYA) Prime enrollment is $180 and $156 for a TYA Standard enrollment.

TRICARE for Life

TRICARE for Life was created as supplemental coverage to Medicare-eligible military retirees by Section 712 of the Floyd D. Spence National Defense Authorization Act for FY2001 (P.L. 106- 398). TRICARE for Life functions as a secondary payer to Medicare, paying out-of-pocket costs for medical services covered under Medicare for beneficiaries who are entitled to Medicare Part A based on age, disability, or end-stage renal disease (ESRD). The beneficiaries are also eligible for medical benefits covered by TRICARE but not by Medicare. Prior to creation of the TRICARE for Life program, coverage for Medicare-eligible individuals was limited to space available care in military treatment facilities. In recognition of the requirement to enroll in Medicare Part B, TRICARE for Life cost-sharing for beneficiaries is limited and there is no enrollment charge.

In order to participate in TRICARE for Life, these TRICARE-eligible beneficiaries must enroll in and pay monthly premiums for Medicare Part B.

TRICARE-eligible beneficiaries who are entitled to Medicare Part A based on age, disability, or ESRD, but decline Part B, lose eligibility for TRICARE benefits.[8] In addition, individuals who choose not to enroll in Medicare Part B upon becoming eligible may elect to do so later during an annual enrollment period; however, the Medicare Part B late enrollment penalty may apply.[9]

7. How Much Does Military Health Care Cost Beneficiaries?

Each TRICARE plan has its own cost-sharing arrangements based upon the sponsor's military status and where the care is received (military treatment facility, network provider, or non-network provider).

Active duty service members receive medical care at no cost. Active duty family members pay nothing out-of-pocket for any type of care unless using the point-of-service option. The point-ofservice option (which allows eligible Prime beneficiaries to pay a fee to access authorized providers for routine or urgent care without a referral) has an annual $300 outpatient care deductible for individual coverage and $600 for family coverage. After the deductible is met, beneficiaries who use the point of service option pay 50% of the TRICARE-allowable charge as a cost-share.

The tables below illustrate selected beneficiary cost-share arrangements.

Table 1. Selected TRICARE Cost-Sharing Features

	TRICARE Prime	TRICARE Extra/Standard
Annual Enrollment Fee	Enrollment is required. There is no enrollment fee for active duty families. Retirees, their families and all others must pay annual enrollment fees to participate. For enrollments in fiscal year 2014, the fee is: Individual: $273.84 per year Family: $547.68 per year	None. Enrollment is not required.
Annual Deductible	No annual deductible unless you are using the point-of-service option: $300/Individual $600/Family Note: Active duty service members can't use the point-of-service option.	Active duty family members (sponsor rank E-4 and below): $50/Individual $100/Family Active duty family members (sponsor rank E-5 and above) : $150/Individual

	TRICARE Prime	TRICARE Extra/Standard
		$300/Family All others: $150/Individual $300/Family Note: The annual deductible is waived for Guard/Reserve family members whose sponsor was activated in support of a contingency operation.
Outpatient Visit	Active duty service members: $0 Active duty family members: $0 All others: $12 per visit Non-network Provider: With Primary Care Manager (PCM) referral: Same as network provider costs Without PCM referral: Point-of-service fees apply Note: Active duty service members may not use the point-of-service option.	Network Provider (Extra option): Active duty family members: 15% of negotiated fee after the annual deductible is met All others: 20% of negotiated fee after the annual deductible is met Non-network Provider (Standard option): Active duty family members: 20% of allowable charges after the annual deductible is met All others: 25% allowable charges after the annual deductible is met
Maximum Annual Out-of-Pocket Charge (Catastrophic Cap)	Active duty families: $1,000 per family, per fiscal year National Guard and Reserve families: $1,000 per family, per fiscal year Retired families (and all others): $3,000 per family, per fiscal year	Same as under Prime.

Source: TRICARE web site: http://www.tricare.mil/Welcome/ComparePlans.aspx
Notes: Current as of October 1, 2013.

8. What Is the Pharmacy Benefits Program?

The Pharmacy Benefits Program is an adjunct to the various TRICARE plan options. Under this program, TRICARE beneficiaries are able to obtain prescription drugs through military treatment facilities, retail drug stores, and a national mail order plan. The Pharmacy Benefit Program is authorized under 10 U.S.C. 1074g.

The Pharmacy Benefits Program is required to maintain a formulary of pharmaceutical agents (hereinafter also referred to as "drugs" or "medications") in the complete range of therapeutic classes. This is known as the "Uniform Formulary." Selection of drugs for inclusion on the formulary is based on the relative clinical and cost effectiveness of the agents in each class.[10] The law further specifies that the formulary is to be maintained and updated by a Pharmacy and Therapeutics Committee whose members are composed of representatives of both military treatment facility pharmacies and health care providers.[11]

The Pharmacy and Therapeutics Committee meets at least quarterly and its minutes are publicly available.[12] A Uniform Formulary Beneficiary Advisory (UFBA) is required to review and comment on formulary recommendations presented by the Pharmacy and Therapeutics Committee prior to those recommendations going to the Executive Director of TRICARE for approval.

The UFBBA is composed of representatives of nongovernmental organizations and associations that represent the views and interests of a large number of eligible covered beneficiaries, contractors responsible for the TRICARE retail pharmacy program, contractors responsible for the national mail-order pharmacy program, and TRICARE network providers.[13]

Prescriptions Filled through Military Treatment Facilities

At a military treatment facility pharmacy, TRICARE beneficiaries may fill prescriptions from any provider, civilian or military, without a copayment. Military treatment facilities are required to stock a subset of the Uniform Formulary known as the "Basic Core Formulary." Additional pharmaceutical agents on the Uniform Formulary may also be carried by individual military treatment facilities in order to meet local requirements. Non-formulary drugs are generally not available through military treatment facilities. Certain Uniform Formulary covered pharmaceuticals, however, may not be carried due to national contracts with pharmaceutical manufactures.[14] DOD's Pharmacoeconomics Center collaborates with the Defense Supply Center Philadelphia (DSCP) in coordination with the Department of Veterans Affairs (VA) Pharmacy Benefits Management Strategic Health Group and the VA National Acquisition Center in Hines, Illinois, in developing contracting strategies and technical evaluation factors for national pharmaceutical contracting initiatives.

Prescriptions Filled through Retail Pharmacies

TRICARE beneficiaries also may fill prescriptions through retail pharmacy drug stores. DOD contracts for a TRICARE pharmacy benefit manager to administer both the retail and mail order options. The services provided by this contractor are known as "TPharm." The current contract, awarded in 2008, is with Express Scripts, Inc. (Express Scripts). Among other things, Express Scripts maintains a national network of retail pharmacies for DOD that beneficiaries may use without having to file a claim for reimbursement. Beneficiaries may also use non-network pharmacies. However, at non-network pharmacies, beneficiaries pay the full price of the medication up front and then file a claim for reimbursement.

DOD requires prescriptions to be filled, when available, with generic drugs. These are defined as those medications approved by the Food and Drug Administration that are clinically the same as brand-name medications. Brand-name drugs that have a generic equivalent are only dispensed after the prescribing provider completes a clinical assessment that indicates the brand-name drug should be used in place of the generic medication and approval is granted by Express Scripts.

Currently, the copayments for non-active duty beneficiaries for a 30-day supply of medicine filled through a network pharmacy are $5 for generic formulary medications, $17 for brand-name formulary medications, and $44 for non-formulary medications, unless medical necessity is established. Copayments for prescriptions filled at non-network pharmacies vary based on the TRICARE plan covering the beneficiary and the type of prescription:

- Active duty service members receive full reimbursement after they file a claim.
- All others enrolled in a TRICARE Prime option pay a 50% cost share after a deductible is met. This deductible is $50 per person and $100 per family per year for service members in pay grades E1–E4 and $150 per person and $300 per family for all other beneficiaries.
- After annual deductibles of $150 per person and $300 per family are met, beneficiaries using Standard/Extra, TRICARE Reserve Select, TRICARE Retired Reserve or TRICARE Young Adult for a 30-day supply pay $17 or 20% of the total cost, whichever is greater, for formulary generic or brand name drugs, and, $44 or 20% of the total cost, whichever is greater, for non-formulary medications.[15]
- Under recent legislation,[16] pharmaceuticals paid for by DOD that are provided by network retail pharmacies to TRICARE beneficiaries are

subject to federal pricing standards. These pricing standards were established under the Veterans Health Care Act of 1992.[17] This act established federal ceiling prices for covered pharmaceuticals, which require a minimum 24% discount off non-federal average manufacturing prices. As a result, the overall growth of retail prescription drug costs for DOD has slowed.[18]

Prescriptions Filled by Mail Order

TRICARE beneficiaries may arrange for home delivery of prescription drugs through the mail by registering with Express Scripts. The copayments for a 90-day supply of medication filled by mail order are currently $13 for brand-name formulary medications, and $43 for non-formulary medications, unless medical necessity is established. Copayments for home delivery of generic drugs were eliminated effective October 1, 2011, as an incentive for beneficiaries to use the home delivery service. DOD negotiates prices with pharmaceutical manufacturers for the drugs dispensed by mail order that are considerably lower than those for drugs dispensed through retail pharmacies. In November 2009, DOD launched a campaign to educate beneficiaries on the benefits of home delivery services. Use of home delivery by TRICARE beneficiaries increased by 17% from FY2009 to FY2011.[19]

Copayment Adjustments

The Secretary of Defense is authorized to set and adjust copayment requirements for the pharmacy program under 10 U.S.C. 1074g; however, Section 712 of the National Defense Authorization Act for FY2013 amended this provision to limit any copayment increases in FY2014 to FY2022 to the percentage by which retirement pay is increased that year.

9. What Is the Extended Care Health Option (ECHO) Program?

The Extended Care Health Option (ECHO) is a program for qualified beneficiaries that supplements TRICARE. It provides benefits that are not covered by TRICARE, such as assistive services, equipment, in-home respite care services and special education for qualifying mental or physical conditions. Qualifying conditions include:

- Diagnosis in an infant or toddler of a neuromuscular developmental condition or other condition expected to precede a diagnosis of moderate or severe mental retardation or serious physical disability;
- Extraordinary physical or psychological conditions causing the beneficiary to be homebound;
- Moderate or severe mental retardation;
- Multiple disabilities, and;
- Severe physical disability.

Access to ECHO benefits requires registration. To use ECHO, qualified beneficiaries must be enrolled in the Exceptional Family Member Program (EFMP) as provided by the sponsor's branch of service and be registered through the ECHO case manager in the applicable TRICARE region. There are no enrollment fees, but there is a monthly cost share based on the sponsor's pay grade. For 2013, monthly costs range from $25 for pay grades E-1 through E-4 to $250 for pay grade O-10. The total TRICARE cost share for all ECHO benefits combined, excluding the ECHO Home Health Care (EHHC) benefit, is $36,000 per covered beneficiary per fiscal year.[20]

EHHC provides medically-necessary skilled services to those ECHO beneficiaries who are homebound and generally require more than 28 to 35 hours per week of home health services or respite care. The EHHC benefit is only available in the United States, District of Columbia, Puerto Rico, the U.S. Virgin Islands, and Guam. Coverage for the EHHC benefit is capped on an annual basis. The cap is limited to the maximum fiscal year amount TRICARE would pay if the beneficiary resided in a skilled nursing facility. This amount is based on the beneficiary's geographic location.

ECHO qualified beneficiaries include:

- Active duty family members;
- Family members of activated National Guard/Reserve members;
- Family members who are covered under the Transitional Assistance Management Program;
- Children or spouses of former service members who are victims of abuse and qualify for the Transitional Compensation Program; and
- Family members of deceased active duty sponsors while they are considered "transitional survivors."

ECHO is authorized under 10 U.S.C. 1079.

10. How Are Priorities for Care in Military Medical Facilities Assigned?

Active duty personnel, military retirees, and their respective dependents are not afforded equal access to care in military medical facilities. Active duty personnel receive top priority access and are "entitled" to health care in a military medical facility (10 U.S.C. 1074).

According to 10 U.S.C. 1076, dependents of active duty personnel are "entitled, upon request, to medical and dental care" on a space-available basis at a military medical facility. 10 U.S.C. 1074 states that "a member or former member of the uniformed services who *is* entitled to retired or retainer pay ... may, upon request, be given medical and dental care in any facility of the uniformed service" on a space-available basis.

This language entitles active duty dependents to medical and dental care subject to space-available limitations. No such entitlement or "right" is provided to retirees or their dependents. Instead, retirees and their dependents may be given medical and dental care, subject to the same space-available limitations. This language gives active duty personnel and their dependents priority in receiving medical and dental care at any facility of the uniformed services over military members entitled to receive retired pay and their dependents. The policy of providing active duty dependents priority over retirees in the receipt of medical and dental care in any facility of the uniformed services has existed in law since at least September 2, 1958 (P.L. 85- 861).

Since the establishment of TRICARE and pursuant to the Defense Authorization Act of FY1996 (P.L. 104-106), DOD has established the following basic priorities (with certain special provisions):

- Priority 1: Active-duty servicemembers;
- Priority 2: Active-duty family members who are enrolled in TRICARE Prime;
- Priority 3: Retirees, their family members and survivors who are enrolled in TRICARE Prime;
- Priority 4: Active-duty family members who are not enrolled in TRICARE Prime; Priority 5: All other eligible persons.

The priority is given to active duty dependents to help them obtain care easily, and thus make it possible for active duty members to perform their military service without worrying about health care for their dependents. This is particularly important for active duty personnel who may be assigned overseas or aboard ship and separated from their dependents. As retirees are not subject to such imposed separations, they are considered to be in a better position to see that their dependents receive care, if care cannot be provided in a military facility. Thus, the role of health care delivery recognizes the unique needs of the military mission. The role of health care in the military is qualitatively different, and, therefore, not necessarily comparable to the civilian sector.

The benefits available to servicemembers or retirees, which require comparatively little or no contributions from the beneficiaries themselves, are considered by some to be a more generous benefit package than is available to civil servants or to most people in the private sector. Retirees may also be eligible to receive medical care at Department of Veterans Affairs (VA) medical facilities.

11. What Are the Long-Term Trends in Defense Health Costs?

Even as the number of active duty personnel in DOD declines over the next few years, costs associated with the military health system are expected to grow. Total military health system costs (excluding TRICARE for Life) increased between FY2009 and FY2011 for inpatient and outpatient services but declined for prescription drugs, due to the FY2008 NDAA requirement that the TRICARE retail pharmacy program be subject to the same pricing standards as other federal agencies.

DOD's FY2013 appropriations request for the Defense Health Program and the Medical Eligible Retiree Health Fund was approximately 7.4% of DOD's total FY2013 appropriations request.[21] The Congressional Budget Office (CBO) projects that the cost of the military health care system will grow from $51 billion in FY2013 (higher than DOD's FY2013 budget request of $47 billion) to $65 billion by FY2017 and $95 billion by FY2030.22 Over the Future Years Defense Plan (FYDP) period from FY2013 to FY2017, CBO's projection has average annual growth of 6.0%, compared with 2.6% in DOD's projection. Over the entire FY2013-FY2030 period, CBO estimates the real (inflation-adjusted) growth rates in cost per user in the military health system would average 5.5% per year for pharmaceuticals, 4.7% for purchased care and contracts, and 3.3% for direct care and administration. Please see Figure 3 and Figure 4 below. Overall, DOD forecasts expect Defense Health

Program costs to increase by 3.4% in FY2014, 3.35% in FY2015, 3.6% in FY2016, and 3.9% in FY2017, in constant FY2013 dollars.[23]

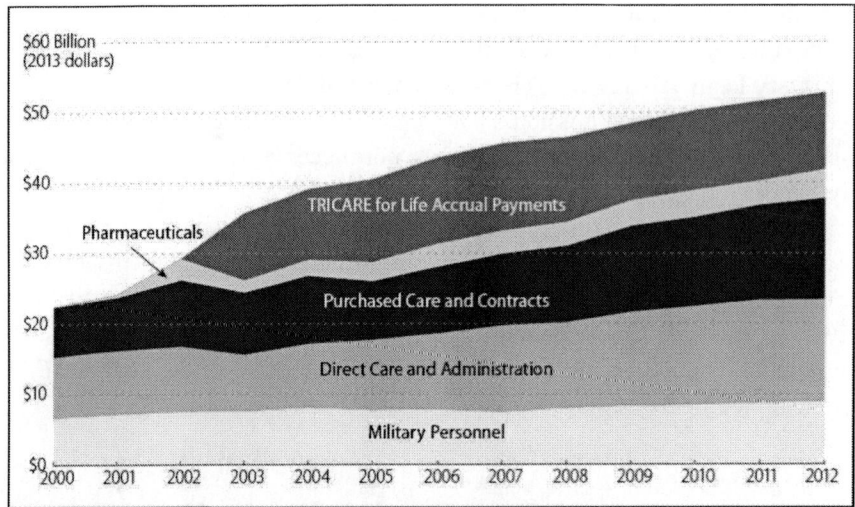

Source: Carla Tighe Murray, Approaches to Reduce Federal Spending on the Defense Health System, Congressional Budget Office, July 31, 2013, p. 3, http://www.cbo.gov/publication/44393.

Figure 3. CBO Depiction of Funding for the MHS, by Category.

This cost growth stems in part from general inflation in the cost of health care, as well as an increasing percentage of care being provided to retirees and their dependents. DOD estimates that care provided to retirees and their dependents will make up over 65% of DOD health care costs by 2015, up from 43% in 1999. A recent CBO analysis concludes that this increasing proportion of retirees participating in TRICARE is driven by "low out-of-pocket expenses for TRICARE beneficiaries (many of whose copayments, deductibles, and maximum annual out-of-pocket payments have remained unchanged or have decreased since the mid-1990s), combined with increased costs of alternative sources of health insurance coverage." In addition, CBO found that TRICARE beneficiaries use both inpatient and outpatient care at rates significantly higher than people with other insurance, due to low out-of-pocket costs and other factors.

DOD proposed new fees and cost-sharing increases for retiree TRICARE plans in their FY2013 budget submission. The new fee proposals were generally based on recommendations by the 2007 Task Force on the Future of Military Health Care. This congressionally created task force found that, "because costs borne by retirees under age 65 have been fixed in dollar terms since 1996, when TRICARE was being established, the portion of medical care costs assumed by these military retirees has declined by a factor of 2-3."[24] Overall, "military health care premiums paid by individual military retirees under age 65 utilizing DOD's most popular plan (TRICARE Prime) have fallen from 11% to 4%" of total health care costs.[25] These proposed cost-sharing increases and new fees were not adopted by the 112th Congress; however, as discussed above in "7. How Much Does Military Health Care Cost Beneficiaries?" above, some increases to pharmacy copayments were provided for in the National Defense Authorization Act for Fiscal Year 2013. The President's 2014 Budget also proposed new fee increases, however, none of these were adopted in the National Defense Authorization Act for Fiscal Year 2014.

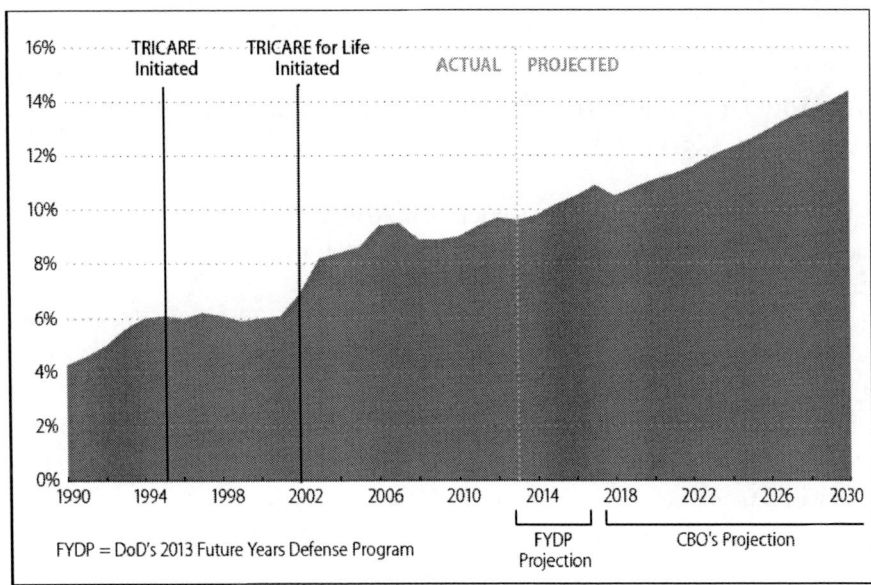

Source: Carla Tighe Murray, Approaches to Reduce Federal Spending on the Defense Health System, Congressional Budget Office, July 31, 2013, p. 2, http://www.cbo.gov/publication/44393.

Figure 4. CBO Depiction of Actual and Projected Costs for Military Health Care as a Share of DoD's Budget, 1990 to 2030.

DOD proposed new fees and cost-sharing increases for retiree TRICARE plans in their FY2013 budget submission. The new fee proposals were generally based on recommendations by the 2007 Task Force on the Future of

Military Health Care. This congressionally created task force found that, "because costs borne by retirees under age 65 have been fixed in dollar terms since 1996, when TRICARE was being established, the portion of medical care costs assumed by these military retirees has declined by a factor of 2-3."[24] Overall, "military health care premiums paid by individual military retirees under age 65 utilizing DOD's most popular plan (TRICARE Prime) have fallen from 11% to 4%" of total health care costs.[25] These proposed cost-sharing increases and new fees were not adopted by the 112th Congress; however, as discussed above in "7. How Much Does Military Health Care Cost Beneficiaries?" above, some increases to pharmacy copayments were provided for in the National Defense Authorization Act for Fiscal Year 2013. The President's 2014 Budget also proposed new fee increases, however, none of these were adopted in the National Defense Authorization Act for Fiscal Year 2014.

12. How Does the Patient Protection and Affordable Care Act Affect TRICARE?

In general, the Patient Protection and Affordable Care Act (ACA)[26] does not directly affect TRICARE administration, health care benefits, eligibility, or cost to beneficiaries.[27]

Section 3110 of the ACA did open a special Medicare Part B enrollment window to enable certain individuals to gain coverage under the TRICARE for Life program.[28]

The ACA also waived the Medicare Part B late enrollment penalty during the 12-month special enrollment period (SEP) for military retirees, their spouses (including widows/widowers), and dependent children who are otherwise eligible for TRICARE and are entitled to Medicare Part A based on disability or end-stage renal disease, but have declined Part B. The ACA required that the Secretary of Defense to identify and notify individuals of their eligibility for the SEP; the Secretary of Health and Human Services (HHS) and the Commissioner for Social Security support these efforts administratively.

Section 3110 of the ACA was amended by the Medicare and Medicaid Extenders Act of 2010[29] to clarify that Section 3110 applies to Medicare Part B elections made on or after the date of enactment of the PPACA, which was on March 23, 2010.

13. How Are Private Health Care Providers Paid?

By law (P.L. 102-396) and Federal Regulation (32 CFR 199.14), health care providers treating TRICARE patients cannot bill for more than 115% of charges authorized by a DOD fee schedule. In some geographic areas, providers have been unwilling to accept TRICARE patients because of the limits on fees that can be charged. DOD has authority to grant exceptions. Statutes (10 U.S.C. 1079(h) and (j)) also require that payment levels for health care services provided under TRICARE be aligned with Medicare's fee schedule "to the extent practicable." Over 90% of TRICARE payment levels are now equivalent to those authorized by Medicare, about 10% are higher, and steps are being taken to adjust some to Medicare levels.

For institutional providers of outpatient services, TRICARE published a final regulation[30] that became effective on May 1, 2009, implementing the TRICARE outpatient prospective payment system (OPPS). Under 10 U.S.C. 1079(j)(2), DOD is required to use Medicare's reimbursement payment system for hospital outpatient services to the extent practicable. Under the OPPS, hospital outpatient services are paid on a rate-per-service basis that varies according to the Ambulatory Payment Classification (APC) group to which the services are assigned. Group services identified by Health Care Procedure Coding System (HCPCS) codes and descriptors within APC groups are the basis for setting payment rates under the hospital OPPS. To receive TRICARE reimbursement under the OPPS, providers must follow all Medicare specific coding requirements, except in those instances where the TRICARE Management Activity (TMA) develops specific APCs for those services that are unique to the TRICARE beneficiary population. For inpatient services, TMA regularly publishes reimbursement schedules through the Federal Register.

14. What Is the Relationship of DOD Health Care to Medicare?

TRICARE and Medicare Payments to Providers and the Sustainable Growth Rate

TRICARE is required to pay healthcare providers "to the extent practicable, in accordance with the same reimbursement rules as apply to payments for similar services"[31] under Medicare. This requirement was added by Section 731 of the National Defense Authorization Act for Fiscal Year 1996.[32]

The Sustainable Growth Rate (SGR) is the statutory method for determining the annual updates to the Medicare physician fee schedule, created in the Balanced Budget Act of 1997.[33] Under the SGR formula, "if [Medicare] expenditures over a period are less than the cumulative spending target for the period, the annual update [to the provider fee schedule] is increased. However, if spending exceeds the cumulative spending target over a certain period, future updates are reduced to bring spending back in line with the target."[34] In other words, if Medicare costs are greater than expected, the provider fees are reduced to bring overall Medicare expenditures down towards expected levels.[35]

Each year since 2002, the SGR system has produced a formula result, "conversion factor" that would reduce reimbursement rates. With the exception of 2002, when a 4.8% decrease was applied, Congress has overridden the SGR formula-driven reductions to provider fee rates through a series of temporary postponements known as "doc fixes."

Most recently, the Pathway for SGR Reform Act of 2013 (§1101 of H.J.Res. 59) overrode the SGR formula-driven reimbursement rates until March 31, 2014. The most recent calculation of the cut in reimbursement rates that would have occurred absent an override was 23.7%.[36]

Although the law requires TRICARE reimbursement rates to be equal to Medicare rates "to the extent practicable," it does permit TRICARE to make exceptions to ensure an adequate network of providers or to eliminate a situation of severely impaired access to care.

Medicare and TRICARE for Life

Active duty military personnel have been fully covered by Social Security and have paid Social Security taxes since January 1, 1957. In 1965, Congress created Medicare under Title 18 of the Social Security Act to provide health insurance to people age 65 and older, regardless of income or medical history. Social Security coverage includes eligibility for health care coverage under Medicare at age 65.

In establishing CHAMPUS in 1966, it was the legislative intent of Congress that retired members of the uniformed services and their eligible dependents be provided with medical care after they retire from the military, usually between their late-30s and mid-40s. However, Congress did not intend that CHAMPUS should replace Medicare as a supplemental benefit to military health care. For this reason, retirees became ineligible to receive CHAMPUS benefits when, at age 65, they become eligible for Medicare.

Many argued that the structure was inherently unfair because retirees lost TRICARE/CHAMPUS benefits at the stage in life when they were increasingly likely to need them. It was argued that military personnel had been promised free medical care for life, not just until age 65. After considerable debate over various options for ensuring medical care to retired beneficiaries, Congress in the Floyd D. Spence National Defense Authorization Act for Fiscal Year 2001[37] provided that, beginning October 1, 2001, TRICARE would pay out-of-pocket costs for services provided under Medicare for beneficiaries over age 64 if they are enrolled in Medicare Part B. This benefit is known as TRICARE for Life (TFL). Disabled persons under age 65 who are entitled to Medicare may continue to receive CHAMPUS benefits as a secondary payer to Medicare Parts A and B (with some restrictions).

The requirement for enrollment in Medicare Part B, which has typical premiums of $104.90 per month in 2013,[38] is a source of concern to some beneficiaries, especially those who did not enroll in Part B when they became 65 and thus must pay significant penalties. Some argue that this requirement is unfair since Part B enrollment was not originally a prerequisite for access to any DOD medical care. On the other hand, waiving the penalty for military retirees could be considered unfair to other Medicare-users who did not enroll in Part B upon turning 65. The Medicare Prescription Drug, Improvement, and Modernization Act[39] (P.L. 108-173), passed in December 2003, waived penalties for military retirees in certain circumstances during an open season in 2004.[40] More recently, the ACA created another special enrollment period. (See question #12).

15. What Medical Benefits Are Available to Reservists?

Reservists and National Guardsmen (members of the "Reserve Component") who are serving on active duty have the same medical benefits as regular military personnel. Reserve personnel while on active duty for training and during weekly or monthly drills also are covered for illnesses incurred while on training or traveling to or from their duty station. In recent years, especially as members of the Reserve Component have had a larger role in combat operations overseas, Congress has broadened the medical benefits available for Reservists. Those who have been notified that they are to be activated are now covered by TRICARE up to 180 days before reporting. Reservists who have served more than 30 days after having been called up for active duty in a contingency operation are eligible for 180 days of TRICARE coverage after the end of their service under the Transitional Assistance Management Program (TAMP). In addition, the TRICARE Reserve Select (TRS) program is an optional program available to Reserve Component members while not activated. To be eligible for TRS, the member must not be on active duty orders, not be covered under the Transitional Assistance Management Program, and not be eligible for or enrolled in the Federal Employees Health Benefits Program. TRS coverage requires payment of monthly premiums (in 2013, $51.62 for individual coverage, $195.81 for member and family coverage).

16. Have Military Personnel Been Promised Free Medical Care for Life?

Some military personnel and former military personnel maintain that they and their dependents were promised "free medical care for life" at the time of their enlistment. Such promises may have been made by military recruiters and in recruiting brochures; however, if they were made, they were not based upon laws or official regulations, which provide only for access to military medical facilities for non-active-duty personnel if space is available as described above. Space was not always available and TRICARE options could involve significant costs to beneficiaries. Rear Admiral Harold M. Koenig, the Deputy Assistant Secretary of Defense for Health Affairs, testified in May 1993: "We have a medical care program for life for our beneficiaries, and it is pretty well defined in the law. That easily gets interpreted to, or reinterpreted into, free medical care for the rest of your life. That is a pretty easy transition for people to make in their thinking, and it is pervasive. We [DOD] spend an incredible amount of effort trying to re-educate people [that] that is not their benefit."[41]

Dr. Stephen C. Joseph, Assistant Secretary of Defense for Health Affairs in April 1998, however, argued that because retirees believe they have had a promise of free care, the government did have an obligation. Joseph did not specify the precise extent of the obligation. The FY1998 Defense Authorization Act (P.L. 105-85) included (in Section 752) a finding that "many retired military personnel believe that they were promised lifetime health care in exchange for 20 or more years of service," and expressed the sense of Congress that "the United States has incurred a moral obligation to provide health care to members and [retired] members of the Armed Services." Further, it is necessary "to provide quality, affordable care to such retirees."

17. What Is the Congressionally Directed Medical Research Program?

Many different entities within the Department of Defense request appropriations for and are funded to conduct a wide range of medical research. Over the last 17 years, Congress has supplemented the DOD appropriations to include additional unrequested funding for specific medical research funding. In 1992, Congress appropriated $25 million for breast cancer research to be managed by DOD's U.S. Army Medical Research and Materiel Command (USAMRMC). The following year, Congress appropriated $210 million to the DOD for extramural, peer-reviewed breast cancer research.

Following this, DOD established the Congressionally Directed Medical Research Programs (CDMRP) within USAMRMC. The Program now manages congressionally directed appropriations totaling $6 billion through FY2010 for research on breast, prostate, and ovarian cancers; neurofibromatosis; military health; chronic myelogenous leukemia; tuberous sclerosis complex; autism; psychological health and traumatic brain injury; amyotrophic lateral sclerosis; Gulf War Illness; deployment-related health research; and other health concerns.[42] This additional, unrequested funding now appears in the Defense Health Program RDT&E appropriation. Conference report language usually includes a table instructing DOD on how to allocate the additional funding to specific diseases and research areas. This guidance is not considered to be an earmark because the funding is used for peer-reviewed, competitively awarded research grants.

Table 2 depicts appropriations for selected CDMRP programs.

Table 2. Appropriation Levels by Fiscal Year (FY) for Selected CDMR Programs, FY2007-FY2013 (in millions of current dollars)

	$FY2007^a$	$FY2008^b$	$FY2009^c$	$FY2010^d$	$FY2011^e$	$FY2012^f$	$FY2013^g$
Amyotrophic Lateral Sclerosis	5	0	5	7.5	8	6.4	7.5
Autism	7.5	6.4	8	8	6.4	5.1	6.0
Bone Marrow Failure	0	0	5	3.75	4	3.2	3.2
Breast Cancer/Breast Cancer Research	127.5	138	150	150	150	120	120

Table 2. (Continued)

	FY2007[a]	*FY2008*[b]	*FY2009*[c]	*FY2010*[d]	*FY2011*[e]	*FY2012*[f]	*FY2013*[g]
Gulf War Illness	0	10	8	8	8	10	20
Lung Cancer	0	0	20	15	12.8	10.2	120
Multiple Sclerosis	0	0	5	4.5	4.8	3.8	5
Neurofibromatosis	10	8	10	13.75	16	12.8	15
Ovarian Cancer	10	10	20	18.75	20	16	20
Peer-Reviewed Cancer	0	0	16	15	16	12.8	15
Peer-Reviewed Medical	0	50	50	50	50	50	50
Peer-Reviewed Orthopedic	0	0	51	22.5	24	30	30
Prostate Cancer	80	80	80	80	80	80	80
Psychological Health/Traumatic Brain Injury	150	0	165	120	100	135.5	135
Spinal Cord Injury	0	0	35	11.25	12	9.6	30
Tuberous Sclerosis	0	4	6	6	6.4	5.1	6

Source: Congressionally Directed Medical Research Program, Annual Reports FY2007–FY2012, Recommendations accompanying the Defense Appropriations Acts.

Notes:

[a] Funds appropriated by P.L. 110-5 (see H.Rept. 109-676 to H.R. 5631, September 25, 2006, pages 248-250), http://www.gpo.gov/fdsys/pkg/CRPT-109hrpt676/pdf/CRPT-109hrpt676.pdf.

[b] Funds appropriated by P.L. 110-116. See Congressional Record, November 6, 2007, p. H13119.

[c] Funds appropriated by Division C of P.L. 110-329. See Congressional Record, September 24, 2008, pp. H9725–H9726.

[d] Funds appropriated by P.L. 111-117. See Congressional Record, December 16, 2009, p. H15319–H15320, http://www.gpo.gov/fdsys/pkg/CREC-2009-12-16/pdf/CREC-2009-12-16-pt1-PgH15007-2.pdf#page=314.

[e] Funds appropriated by P.L. 112-10. See House Rules Committee' tables accompanying H.R. 1473, pp. 53-54, http://rules.house.gov/Media/file/FY11-Defense-Department-Base-tables.pdf.

[f] Funds appropriated by P.L. 112-74 (H.R. 2055). See House Rules Committee's tables accompanying H.R. 2055, 92A, p. 282, http://rules.house.gov/Media/ file/PDF_112j/legislativetext/H.R.2055crSOM/psConference%20Div%20A%20-%20SOM%20OCR.pdf.

[g] Funds appropriated by P.L. 113-6 (H.R. 933). Figures not adjusted for sequestration reductions of 7.95%. See Senate Explanation Statement, p. S1515 at

http://www.gpo.gov/fdsys/pkg/CREC-2013-03-11/pdf/CREC2013-03-11-pt1-PgS1287.pdf#page=1.

The CDMRP website (http://cdmrp.army.mil/) also provides specific descriptions and funding histories of the different research programs.

18. Other Frequently Asked Questions

Does TRICARE Cover Abortion?

10 U.S.C. 1093 provides that "Funds available to the Department of Defense may not be used to perform abortions except where the life of the mother would be endangered if the fetus were carried to term or in a case in which the pregnancy is the result of an act of rape or incest."[43]

Does DOD Use Animals in Medical Research or Training?

Yes. DOD policy is that live animals will not be used for training and education except where, after exhaustive analysis, no alternatives are available. Currently approved uses include pre-deployment training for medical personnel and include infant intubation (ferrets); microsurgery (rodents); and combat trauma training (goats and swine).

End Notes

[1] http://www.health.mil/

[2] Department of Defense, Third Submission unders Section 731 of the National Defense Authorization Act for Fiscal year 2013: Plan for Reform of the Administration of the Military Health System, October 25, 2013, pp. 1-6, http://www.tricare.mil/tma/congressionalinformation/downloads/Military%20Health%20System%20Governance%20Reform%20Report.pdf.

[3] Department of Defense, FY 2014 Budget Request Overview, April 2013, pp. 5-3, Figure 5-1, http://comptroller.defense.gov/defbudget/fy2014/FY2014_Budget_Request_Overview_Book.pdf.

[4] P.L. 106-398.

[5] Department of Defense, Fiscal Year 2011 Medicare-Eligible Retiree Health Care Fun Audited Financial Statements, November 7, 2011, p. 5, http://comptroller.defense.gov/cfs/fy2011/12_Medicare_Eligible_Retiree_Health_Care_Fund/Fiscal_Year_2011_Medicare_Eligible_Retiree_Health_Care_Fund_Financial_Statements_and_Notes.pdf.

[6] P.L. 84-569.

[7] P.L 89-614.

[8] 10 U.S.C. §1086(d).

[9] CRS Report R40082, Medicare: Part B Premiums, by Patricia A. Davis.
[10] 10 U.S.C. 1074g(a)(2)(A).
[11] 10 U.S.C. 1074g(b).
[12] Available at the Department of Defense Pharmacoeconomic Center web site: http://www.pec.ha.osd.mil/.
[13] ibid.
[14] Office of the Assistant Secretary of Defense (Health Affairs), Memorandum subject "TRICARE Pharmacy Benefit Program Formulary Management" dated December 22, 2004. Accessed February 27, 2013, at http://pec.ha.osd.mil/P&T/PDF/04-032.pdf.
[15] TRICARE web site accessed February 26, 2013, http://www.tricare.mil/pharmacycosts.
[16] Section 703 of the National Defense Authorization Act for Fiscal Year 2008 (P.L. 110-181).
[17] P.L. 102-585, codified at 38 U.S.C. 8126.
[18] Department of Defense, "Evaluation of the TRICARE Program, Fiscal Year 2012 Report to Congress," March 19, 2012, p. 75. Accessed February 26, 2013, at http://www.tricare.mil/tma/congressionalinformation/downloads/TRICARE%20Evaluation%20Report%20-%20FY12.pdf.
[19] Department of Defense, "Evaluation of the TRICARE Program, Fiscal Year 2012 Report to Congress," March 19, 2012, p. 74. Accessed February 26, 2013, at http://www.tricare.mil/tma/congressionalinformation/downloads/TRICARE%20Evaluation%20Report%20-%20FY12.pdf.
[20] For additional information please see the ECHO web page at http://www.tricare.mil/echo.
[21] Comptroller, Department of Defense. National Defense Budget Estimates for FY2013, March 2012. Table 3-1, Reconciliation of Authorization, Appropriation, TOA and BA, by Program, by Appropriation. pp. 36-44, http://comptroller.defense.gov/defbudget/fy2013/FY13_Green_Book.pdf.
[22] Congressional Budget Office, Long Term Implications of the 2013 Future Years Defense Program, p. 21, http://www.cbo.gov/sites/default/files/cbofiles/attachments/07-11-12-FYDP_forPosting_0.pdf.
[23] Comptroller, Department of Defense. National Defense Budget Estimates for FY2013, March 2012. Table 5-5, Department of Defense Deflators–TOA. p. 60, http://comptroller.defense.gov/defbudget/fy2013/ FY13_Green_Book.pdf.
[24] Department of Defense, subcommittee of the Defense Health Board, "Report of the Task Force on the Future of Military Health Care," December 2007, p. ES10, http://www.dcoe.health.mil/Content/Navigation/Documents/103-06-2-Home-Task_Force_FINAL_RE PORT_122007.pdf.
[25] Department of Defense, subcommittee of the Defense Health Board, "Report of the Task Force on the Future of Military Health Care," December 2007, p. 92, http://www.dcoe.health.mil/Content/Navigation/Documents/103-06-2-Home-Task_Force_FINAL_REPORT_122007.pdf.
[26] P.L. 111-148.
[27] CRS Report R41198, TRICARE and VA Health Care: Impact of the Patient Protection and Affordable Care Act (ACA), by Sidath Viranga Panangala and Don J. Jansen.
[28] §3110 of PPACA, P.L. 111-148.
[29] §201, P.L. 111-309.
[30] Department of Defense, "TRICARE: Outpatient Hospital Prospective Payment System (OPPS); Delay of Effective Date and Additional Opportunity for Public Comment," 74 Federal Register 6228, February 6, 2009.
[31] 10 U.S.C. 1079.

[32] P.L. 104-106.
[33] P.L. 105-33.
[34] See §1848 of the Social Security Act codified at 42 U.S.C. 1395w–4.
[35] For more information on the SGR please see: CRS Report R40907, Medicare Physician Payment Updates and the Sustainable Growth Rate (SGR) System, by Jim Hahn and Janemarie Mulvey.
[36] Congressional Budget Office, Medicare's, December 6, 2013, p. Note a., http://www.cbo.gov/sites/default/files/cbofiles/attachments/2013%20SGR%20Options%20-%20Final%20 Rule.pdf.
[37] P.L. 106-398.
[38] CRS Report R40082, Medicare: Part B Premiums, by Patricia A. Davis.
[39] P.L. 108-173.
[40] See out-of-print CRS Report RS21731, Medicare: Part B Premium Penalty, by Jennifer O'Sullivan, available upon request.
[41] U.S. Congress, House of Representatives, Committee on Armed Services, Military Forces and Personnel Subcommittee, 103rd Congress, 1st session, National Defense Authorization Act for Fiscal Year 1994—H.R. 2401 and Oversight of Previously Authorized Programs, Hearings, H.A.S.C. No. 103-13, April 27, 28, May 10, 11, and 13, 1993, p. 505.
[42] Department of Defense, Congressionally Directed Medical Research Program: FY 2008 Annual Report, September 30, 2008, pp. 1-2, http://cdmrp.army.mil/annreports/2008annrep/default.htm.
[43] The clause "or in a case in which the pregnancy is the result of an act of rape or incest" was added by Section 704 of the National Defense Authorization Act for Fiscal Year 2013.

In: Military Medical Care ...
Editor: Adam Seward

ISBN: 978-1-63117-531-2
© 2014 Nova Science Publishers, Inc.

Chapter 2

HEALTH CARE FOR VETERANS: ANSWERS TO FREQUENTLY ASKED QUESTIONS[*]

Sidath Viranga Panangala and Erin Bagalman

SUMMARY

The Veterans Health Administration (VHA), within the Department of Veterans Affairs (VA), operates the nation's largest integrated health care delivery system, provides care to more than 5.5 million veteran patients, and employs more than 258,000 full-time equivalent employees.

Eligibility and Enrollment. Contrary to claims concerning promises of "free health care for life," not every veteran is automatically entitled to medical care from the VA. Eligibility for VA health care is based primarily on veteran status resulting from military service. Generally, veterans must also meet minimum service requirements; however, exceptions are made for veterans discharged due to service-connected disabilities, members of the Reserve and National Guard (under certain circumstances), and returning combat veterans. The VA categorizes veterans into eight Priority Groups, based on factors such as service-connected disabilities and income (among others). Dependents, caregivers, and survivors of certain veterans are eligible for the Civilian

---

[*] This is an edited, reformatted and augmented version of a Congressional Research Service publication, CRS Report for Congress R42747, from www.crs.gov, prepared for Members and Committees of Congress, dated August 1, 2013.

Health and Medical Program of the Department of Veterans Affairs (CHAMPVA), which reimburses non-VA providers or facilities for their medical care.

Medical Benefits. All enrolled veterans are offered a standard medical benefits package, which includes (but is not limited to) inpatient and outpatient medical services, pharmaceuticals, durable medical equipment, and prosthetic devices.

For female veterans, the VA provides gender-specific care, such as gynecological care, breast and reproductive oncology, infertility treatment, maternity care, and care for conditions related to military sexual trauma. Under current regulations, the VA is not authorized to provide, or cover the costs of, in vitro fertilization, abortion counseling, abortions, or medication to induce abortions.

Generally the VA provides audiology and eye care services (including preventive services and routine vision testing) for all enrolled veterans, but eyeglasses and hearing aids are provided only to veterans meeting certain criteria. Eligibility for VA dental care is limited and differs significantly from eligibility for medical care. For veterans with service-connected disabilities who meet certain criteria, the VA provides short- and long-term nursing care, respite, and end-oflife care.

Under certain circumstances, the VA may reimburse non-VA providers for health care services rendered to VA-enrolled veterans on a fee-for-service basis. Such Fee Basis Care may include outpatient care, inpatient care, emergency care, medical transportation, and dental services.

Costs to Veterans and Insurance Collections. While enrolled veterans do not pay premiums for VA care, some veterans are required to pay copayments for medical services and outpatient medications related to the treatment of nonservice-connected conditions. Copayment amounts vary by Priority Group and type of service (e.g., inpatient versus outpatient). The VA has the authority to bill most health care insurers for nonservice-connected care; any insurer's payment received by the VA is used to offset "dollar for dollar" a veteran's VA copayment responsibility. The VA is statutorily prohibited from receiving Medicare payments (with a narrow exception).

INTRODUCTION

The Veterans Health Administration (VHA), within the Department of Veterans Affairs (VA), operates the nation's largest integrated direct health care delivery system, provides care to more than 5.5 million unique veteran patients,[1] and employs more than 258,000 full-time equivalent employees.[2]

While Medicare, Medicaid, and the Children's Health Insurance Program (CHIP) are also publicly funded programs, most health care services under these programs are delivered by private providers in private facilities. In contrast, the VA health care system could be categorized as a veteran-specific national health care system, in the sense that the federal government owns the medical facilities and employs the health care providers.[3]

This report provides responses to frequently asked questions about health care provided to veterans through the VHA. It is intended to serve as a quick reference to provide easy access to information. Where applicable, it provides the legislative background pertaining to the question.

ENROLLMENT IN VA HEALTH CARE

Can All Veterans Enroll in VA Health Care?

Not every veteran is automatically eligible to enroll in VA health care, contrary to numerous claims made concerning "promises" to military personnel and veterans with regard to "free health care for life."[4]

Eligibility for enrollment in VA health care has evolved over time. Prior to eligibility reform in 1996, all veterans were technically eligible for some care; however, the actual provision of care was based on available resources.[5]

The Veterans' Health Care Eligibility Reform Act of 1996 (P.L. 104-262) established two eligibility categories and required VHA to manage the provision of hospital care and medical services through an enrollment system based on a system of priorities.[6] (See the *Appendix* for the criteria for the Priority Groups.) P.L. 104-262 authorized the VA to provide all needed hospital care and medical services to veterans with service-connected disabilities;[7] former prisoners of war; veterans exposed to toxic substances and environmental hazards such as Agent Orange; veterans whose attributable income and net worth are not greater than an established "means test"; and veterans of World War I. These veterans are generally known as "higher priority" or "core" veterans.[8] The other category of veterans are those with no service-connected disabilities and with attributable incomes above an established "means test."

P.L. 104-262 also authorized the VA to establish a patient enrollment system to manage access to VA health care. As stated in the report language accompanying P.L. 104-262,

[t]he Act would direct the Secretary, in providing for the care of 'core' veterans, to establish and operate a system of annual patient enrollment and require that veterans be enrolled in a manner giving relative degrees of preference in accordance with specified priorities. At the same time, it would vest discretion in the Secretary to determine the manner in which such enrollment system would operate.[9]

Furthermore, P.L. 104-262 was clear in its intent that the provision of health care to veterans was dependent upon available resources. The committee report accompanying P.L. 104-262 states that the provision of hospital care and medical services would be provided to "the extent and in the amount provided in advance in appropriations Acts for these purposes. Such language is intended to clarify that these services would continue to depend upon discretionary appropriations."[10]

Which Veterans Can Enroll in VA Health Care?

Enrollment in VA health care is based primarily on veteran status (i.e., previous military service), service-connected disability,[11] and income.[12]

Generally, veteran status is established by (1) active duty service in the military, naval, or air service; (2) satisfying a minimum period of duty;[13] and (3) receiving an other than dishonorable discharge or release.[14] Exact requirements for enrollment eligibility depend on various criteria, such as when and in which component (i.e., active, Reserves, or National Guard) the veteran served. See below for questions and answers about returning combat veterans and members of the Reserves and National Guard.

Is Enrollment Different for Returning Combat Veterans?

Veterans returning from combat operations are eligible to enroll in VA health care for five years from the date of their most recent discharge without having to demonstrate a service-connected disability or satisfy an income requirement. Veterans who enroll under this extended enrollment authority continue to be enrolled even after the five-year eligibility period ends.

This special period of enrollment eligibility for VA health care was first established in 1998 and was expanded in 2007. In 1998, Congress, responding to the growing concerns of Persian Gulf War veterans' undiagnosed illnesses, passed the Veterans Programs Enhancement Act of 1998 (P.L. 105-368), entitling a veteran who served on active duty in a theater of combat operations during a period of war after the Persian Gulf War to be eligible to enroll in VA health care during a two-year period following the date of discharge.

In 2007, the National Defense Authorization Act (NDAA), FY2008 (P.L. 110-181) extended the period of enrollment eligibility for VA health care from two to five years for veterans who served in a theater of combat operations after November 11, 1998.[15] If returning veterans do not enroll during this five-year enrollment window (from the date of discharge), future applications for enrollment will be evaluated according to the Priority Group classifications described in the *Appendix*. For this reason, the VA encourages veterans to take advantage of the enhanced enrollment period.

Is Enrollment Different for Members of the Reserves?

When not activated to full-time federal service, members of the Reserve components have limited eligibility for VA health care services.

Similar to regular active duty servicemembers, members of the Reserve components may be eligible for enrollment for VA health care based on veteran status (i.e., previous military service), service-connected disability,[16] and income.

Reservists achieve veteran status and are exempt from the 24-month minimum duty requirement (as described above) if they (1) were called to active duty, (2) completed the term for which they were called, and (3) were granted an other-than-dishonorable discharge.

Members of the Reserve components may be granted service-connection for any injury they incurred or aggravated in the line of duty while attending inactive duty training assemblies, annual training, active duty for training, or while going directly to or returning directly from such duty. In addition, Reserve component servicemembers may be granted service-connection for a heart attack or stroke if such an event occurs during these same periods. The granting of service-connection makes them eligible to receive care from the VA for those conditions.

Is Enrollment Different for Members of the National Guard?

When not activated to full-time federal service, members of the National Guard have limited eligibility for VA health care services.

Similar to regular active duty servicemembers, members of the National Guard may be eligible for enrollment in VA health care based on veteran status (i.e., previous military service), service-connected disability,[17] and income. National Guard members achieve veteran status and are exempt from the 24-month minimum duty requirement (as described above) if they (1) were called to active duty by federal executive order, (2) completed the term for which they were called, and (3) were granted an other than dishonorable discharge.

National Guard members are not granted service-connection for any injury, heart attack, or stroke that occurs while performing duty ordered by a governor for state emergencies or activities.[18]

How Do Veterans Enroll in VA Health Care?

To receive VA health care, most veterans must enroll by completing and submitting the VA's Application for Health Benefits (VA Form 10-10EZ).[19]

The following eight-step VA health care enrollment process is illustrated in *Figure 1:*

1) A veteran may apply for enrollment at any time of year by submitting the application for enrollment (online, in person, by mail, or by fax) to a VA health care facility. The application form includes information about the veteran's military service, demographics, and (as applicable) financial status.
2) Upon receipt of the enrollment application, the VA health care facility enters the information into the Veterans Health Information Systems and Technology Architecture (VistA) system, which creates an electronic record for the veteran. (If the enrollment application is submitted in person, a preliminary eligibility determination is typically provided at the time of application.)
3) The VistA system transmits the veteran's application information to the VA's centralized Eligibility and Enrollment System.
4) The VA's centralized Eligibility and Enrollment System establishes the veteran's record and queries the Veterans Benefits Administration (VBA) records.
5) The VBA returns information about the veteran's military status and/or compensation and pension benefits.
6) The VA's centralized Eligibility and Enrollment System verifies the veteran's enrollment eligibility and shares these data with VistA. (If the enrollment system is unable to determine eligibility, it alerts the veteran's local VA medical center to take further action.)

7) When a determination has been made, the VA's centralized Eligibility and Enrollment System sends the veteran a letter with that information.
8) The veteran receives the letter from the VA.

The VA developed this enrollment process pursuant to the Veterans' Health Care Eligibility Reform Act of 1996 (P.L. 104-262), which required the establishment of a national enrollment system to manage the delivery of veterans' inpatient and outpatient medical care. Congress created the new eligibility standard to "ensure that medical judgment rather than legal criteria will determine when care will be provided and the level at which care will be furnished."[20]

The VA classifies veterans into eight enrollment Priority Groups based on an array of factors, including (but not limited to) service-connected disabilities or exposures,[21] prisoner of war (POW) status, receipt of a Purple Heart or Medal of Honor, and income. (The criteria for each Priority Group are summarized in the *Appendix*.) Once a veteran is enrolled in the VA health care system, the veteran remains in the system and does not have to reapply for enrollment annually. However, those veterans who have been enrolled in Priority Group 5 based on income must submit a new VA Form 10-10EZ annually with updated financial information demonstrating inability to defray the expenses of necessary care.[22]

Are Veterans' Family Members Eligible for VA Health Care?

Veterans 'family members are not eligible for enrollment in VA health care services. However, certain dependents and survivors may receive reimbursement from the VA for some medical expenses.

The Civilian Health and Medical Program of the Department of Veterans Affairs (CHAMPVA) pays for health care services to dependents and survivors of certain veterans. It is primarily a feefor-service program that provides reimbursement for most medical care that is provided by non-VA providers or facilities. On May 5, 2010, President Barack Obama signed into law the Caregivers and Veterans Omnibus Health Services Act of 2010 (P.L. 111-163), which expanded the CHAMPVA program to include the primary family caregiver of an eligible veteran who has no other form of health insurance, including Medicare and Medicaid.23 Health care services provided include counseling, training, and mental health services for the primary family caregiver.

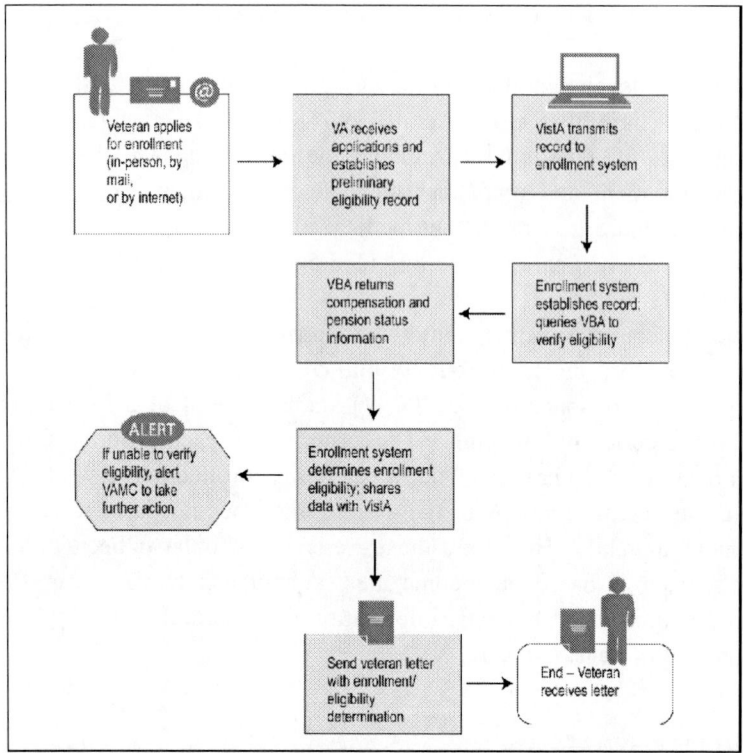

Source: Institute of Medicine, Returning Home from Iraq and Afghanistan: Preliminary Assessment of Readjustment Needs of Veterans, Service Members, and Their Families, 2010, p. 124, adapted by Congressional Research Service.

Notes: VistA = Veterans Health Information Systems and Technology Architecture; VBA = Veterans Benefits Administration; VAMC = VA Medical Center.

Figure 1. VA Health Care Enrollment Process.

MEDICAL BENEFITS

What Are the Standard Medical Benefits?

The VA offers all enrolled veterans a standard medical benefits package that includes (among other things) inpatient care, outpatient care, and prescription drugs.

The VA's standard medical benefits package includes a broad spectrum of inpatient, outpatient, and preventive medical services, such as the following:

- medical, surgical, and mental health care, including care for substance abuse;
- prescription drugs, including over-the-counter drugs, and medical and surgical supplies available under the VA national formulary system;
- durable medical equipment and prosthetic and orthotic devices, including hearing aids and eyeglasses (subject to limitations);[24]
- home health services, hospice care, palliative care, and institutional respite care;
- noninstitutional adult day health care and noninstitutional respite care; and
- periodic medical exams, among other services.[25]

The medical benefits package does not include the following:

- abortions and abortion counseling;
- in vitro fertilization;
- drugs, biologicals, and medical devices not approved by the Food and Drug Administration (FDA), unless the treating medical facility is conducting formal clinical trials under an Investigational Device Exemption (IDE) or an Investigational New Drug (IND) application, or the drugs, biologicals, or medical devices are prescribed under a compassionate use exemption;
- gender alterations;
- hospital and outpatient care for a veteran who is either a patient or inmate in an institution of another government agency if that agency has a duty to give such care or services; and
- membership in spas and health clubs.[26]

Does the VA Provide Gender-Specific Services for Women?

The VA's standard medical benefits package addresses the health care needs of enrolled female veterans by providing (directly or through access to non-VA providers) gynecological care, maternity care, infertility, breast and reproductive oncology, and care for conditions related to military sexual trauma (MST), among other services.

In addition, the Caregivers and Veterans Omnibus Health Services Act of 2010 (P.L. 111-163) authorized the VA to provide certain health care services to a newborn child of a female veteran receiving maternity care furnished by the VA. Health care for the newborn will be authorized for a maximum of seven days after the birth of the child if the veteran delivered the child in a VA facility or in another facility pursuant to a VA contract for maternity services.

Under current regulations, the VA is not authorized to provide or cover the cost of in vitro fertilization (IVF), abortions, abortion counseling, or medication to induce an abortion (e.g., mifepristone, also known as RU-486).[27]

Does the VA Provide Dental Care?

Eligibility for dental care is extremely limited, and differs significantly from eligibility requirements for medical care.

For VA dental care eligibility, enrolled veterans are categorized into classes, which form the basis for the scope of dental treatment provided. *Table 1* describes the eligibility criteria and scope of treatment for VA-provided dental care.

Table 1. Eligibility Criteria and Scope of Treatment for VA Dental Care

Classification	Eligibility Criteria	Scope of Treatment Provided
Class I	Veteran has a service-connected compensable (disability compensation paid) dental condition	Any necessary dental treatment to maintain or restore oral health and masticatory function, including repeat care
Class II	Veteran has a service-connected noncompensable dental condition (not subject to disability compensation) shown to have been in existence at the time of discharge or release from active duty service, which took place after September 30, 1981, if: The veteran served at least 180 days (or 90 days if a veteran of the Gulf War era), and The veteran's DD214[a] does not bear certification that the veteran was provided,	A one-time course of dental treatment of the service-connected noncompensable dental condition

Classification	Eligibility Criteria	Scope of Treatment Provided
	within 90 days immediately prior to discharge or release, a complete dental examination (including dental x-rays) and all appropriate dental treatment indicated by the examination to be needed, and Application for treatment is received within 180 days of discharge	
Class II (a)	Veteran has a service-connected noncompensable dental condition or disability determined as resulting from combat wounds or service trauma	Any necessary dental treatment for the correction of the service-connected condition. Generally, a Dental Trauma Rating or VA Regional Office Rating Decision letter identifies the tooth/teeth eligible for care.
Class II(b)	Veteran is homeless or are otherwise enrolled in certain VA-sponsored rehabilitation programs	A one-time course of dental treatment
Class II(c)	Veteran is a former prisoner of war (POW)	Any necessary dental treatment to maintain or restore oral health and masticatory function, including repeat care
Class III	Veteran has a nonservice-connected dental disability professionally determined to be aggravating a service-connected medical condition	A one-time course of dental treatment to treat only the oral condition that is directly impacting the management of the serviceconnected medical condition. Eligibility for each new course of dental treatment is a based on a new dental evaluation.
Class IV	Veteran whose service-connected disabilities have been rated at 100% or who is receiving the 100% rating by reason of individual unemployability.	Any necessary dental treatment to maintain or restore oral health and masticatory function, including repeat care
Class V	Veteran who is approved for VA vocational rehabilitation training and who requires dental treatment to participate in the training	Dental care to the extent needed to meet any of the following goals: 1. make possible his or her entrance into a rehabilitation program;

Table 1. (Continued)

Classification	Eligibility Criteria	Scope of Treatment Provided
		2. achieve the goals of the veteran's vocational rehabilitation program; 3. prevent interruption of a rehabilitation program; 4. hasten the return to a rehabilitation program of a veteran in interrupted or leave status; 5. hasten the return to a rehabilitation program of a veteran placed in discontinued status because of a dental condition; 6. secure and adjust to employment during the period of employment assistance; or 7. enable the veteran to achieve maximum independence in daily living
Class VI	Veteran scheduled for admission to VA medical center or otherwise receiving care and services, if dental care is reasonably necessary to the provision of such care and services, that is, a dental condition is complicating a medical condition currently under treatment. (Examples: patients scheduled for cardiac surgery, knee, hip, joint replacement surgery, or organ transplant surgery may receive pre-bed care to eliminate dental infection prior to their surgery to help insure successful medical treatment)	A one-time course of dental treatment to treat conditions that directly impact the management of the nonservice-connected medical condition

Source: 38 C.F.R. §§17.160-162 and Department of Veterans Affairs, Veterans Health Administration, Criteria and Standards for Dental Program, VHA Handbook 1130.01, December 25, 2008.

[a] When servicemembers separate from active military service, they each receive a certificate of release or discharge from active duty, known as a DD-214. The DD-214 provides the member and the service with a concise record of a period of service with the Armed Forces at the time of the member's separation, discharge,

or change in military status (reserve/active duty). In addition, the form serves as an authoritative source of information for both governmental agencies and the Armed Forces for purposes of employment, benefit, and reenlistment eligibility, respectively.

The Caregivers and Veterans Omnibus Health Services Act of 2010 (P.L. 111-163) authorized the VHA to conduct a three-year pilot program to assess the feasibility and advisability of providing private, premium-based dental insurance coverage to eligible veterans and certain survivors and dependents. Generally, survivors and dependents that would qualify for the program will be Civilian Health and Medical Program of the VA (CHAMPVA) beneficiaries. Under the three-year pilot program, the VHA would contract with qualified dental insurance carriers that will provide dental insurance and administer all aspects of the dental insurance plan. The VHA would administer the contract with the private insurer and verify eligibility of veterans, survivors, and dependents.[28]

Does the VA Provide Hearing Aids and Eyeglasses?

Generally, the VA provides audiology and eye care services (including preventive care services and routine vision testing) for all enrolled veterans. The VA does not provide hearing aids or eye glasses for normally occurring hearing or vision loss.

Hearing aids and eyeglasses are provided to the following veterans:[29]

- Veterans with any compensable service-connected disability.
- Veterans who are former prisoners of war (POWs).
- Veterans who were awarded a Purple Heart.
- Veterans receiving compensation for an injury, or an aggravation of an injury, that occurred as the result of VA treatment.
- Veterans in receipt of an increased pension based on being permanently housebound and in need of regular aid and attendance.
- Veterans with hearing or vision impairment resulting from diseases or the existence of another medical condition for which the veteran is receiving care or services from VA, or which resulted from treatment of that medical condition (e.g., stroke, polytrauma, traumatic brain injury, diabetes, multiple sclerosis, vascular disease, geriatric chronic illnesses, toxicity from drugs, ocular photosensitivity from drugs,

cataract surgery, and/or other surgeries performed on the eye, ear, or brain resulting in a vision or hearing impairment).
- Veterans with significant functional or cognitive impairment evidenced by deficiencies in the ability to perform activities of daily living.[30]
- Veterans who have hearing and/or vision impairment severe enough that it interferes with their ability to participate actively in their own medical treatment and to reduce the impact of dual sensory impairment (combined hearing and vision loss).

Does the VA Provide Long-Term Care?

The VA provides long-term care services (including residential, home-based, and community-based care) for veterans meeting specified criteria, which may include service-connected conditions and the need for such care.

The Veterans Millennium Healthcare and Benefits Act (P.L. 106-117) requires the VA to provide nursing home services to all enrolled veterans who are 70% or more service-connected disabled, or 60% or more service-connected disabled and unemployable and in need of such care, or who are service-connected for a condition that makes such care necessary.[31] The VA meets the requirements of P.L. 106-117 by providing short- and long-term nursing care, respite, and end-oflife care through three different settings: Community Living Centers (CLCs) located on VA medical campuses; contracted care in Community Nursing Homes (CNH); and through the State Veterans Nursing Home (SVNH) program. Under the SVNH program, the VA subsidizes state-operated, long-term care facilities for veterans through a grant and per diem program in states that have petitioned the VA to build and operate a SVNH. The SVNH program primarily provides long-stay, maintenance-level care. Each SVNH is owned and operated by its host state; however, approximately two-thirds of new construction costs and about one-third of per diem costs are provided by the VA. For those veterans who are 70% or more service-connected disabled and reside in a SVNH, the VA provides the full cost of care.

The VA provides a range of non-institutional home and community based services for veterans, which include the following:

- Skilled Home Care—the Purchased Skilled Home Care Program (formerly known as fee basis home care) is a professional home care service that is purchased from private-sector providers by every VA medical center. A VA primary care provider must recommend Skilled Home Care in order for a veteran to receive it. The professional home care services program covers mostly nursing services, including medical care, social services, occupational therapy, physical therapy, skilled nursing care, and speech and language pathology.

- Home Based Primary Care—This program (formerly known as Hospital Based Home Care) began in 1970 and provides medical care to chronically ill or disabled veterans in their own homes through an interdisciplinary treatment team. These services are paid for by the VA and provided by VA personnel.
- Veteran-Directed Home & Community Based Care—The VA partners with federal Area Agencies on Aging to purchase needed services. This program allows the veteran to decide on a case mix of services to best meet care needs and those of the caregiver.
- Spinal Cord Injury/Disorders Bowel & Bladder Care—These programs provide specialized home care services for veterans with spinal cord injuries and related disorders. Services include respite care, long-term care, bowel and bladder care, and caregiver education to veterans.
- Homemaker/Home Health Aide—This program began in 1993 and provides assistance with personal care and related support services for veterans in their own homes through the homemaker/home health aide (H/HHA) benefit. H/HHA services may include assistance with activities of daily living (ADLs), as well as instrumental activities of daily living (IADLs).32 Eligibility for the H/HHA program is based on a clinical judgment by the H/HHA Coordinator and interdisciplinary team that determines if the veteran would, in the absence of H/HHA services, require nursing home equivalent care. The VA pays for these services. H/HHA services are provided by contracted providers. H/HHAs are personnel who are trained and have completed a competency evaluation, and are placed under the general supervision of a nurse.
- Community Residential Care (CRC)33—CRC is a form of enriched housing that provides health care supervision to eligible veterans not in need of hospital or nursing home care, but who, because of medical and psychiatric and/or psychosocial limitations, as determined through a statement of needed care, are not able to live independently

and have no suitable family or significant others to provide the needed supervision and supportive care. CRCs currently encompass
- assisted living facilities;
- personal care homes;
- family care homes;
- psychiatric community residential care homes; and
- medical foster homes.

In general, each of the settings listed above must provide room, board, assistance with Activities of Daily Living (ADL), and supervision as determined on an individual basis. The individual veteran makes the final choice of facility, and the cost of residential care is financed by the veteran's own resources. However, placement in residential settings is subject to inspection and approval by the appropriate VA medical center.

Table 2. VA Reimbursement for Emergency Care

Service-Connected	Nonservice-Connected
The VA is required to pay or reimburse veterans for medical expenses incurred in non-VA facilities when all three of the following conditions apply:[a] (1) Delay would have been hazardous to the life or health of the veteran. (2) VA or other federal facilities were not feasibly available (or treatment had been refused). (3) The care was provided for: • a service-connected disability, • a nonservice-connected disability aggravating[a] • service-connected disability, or • any disability of a veteran whose service-connected • disability is total and permanent in nature.	The VA is required to pay or reimburse veterans for medical expenses incurred in non-VA facilities when all four of the following conditions apply: (1) Delay would have been hazardous to the life or health of the veteran. (2) VA or other federal facilities were not feasibly available. (3) The veteran has either: • no health coverage (e.g., private health insurance or Medicare) or • coverage that would only partially pay for the emergency treatment.[b] (4) In cases where the care was provided for a condition caused by an accident or work-related injury, all claims against a third party for payment have been exhausted without success.

Source: CRS Summary of 38 U.S.C. §1728 and 38 U.S.C. §1725.

[a] Prior to the enactment of the Veterans' Mental Health and Other Care Improvements Act of 2008 (P.L. 110-387), the VA was not required to reimburse the non-VA facility for the cost of care after the point of stabilization. P.L. 110-387 mandated that the VA reimburse or pay for the reasonable value of treatment for any veteran

who meets above eligibility criteria and defined "emergency treatment" as continuing until the veteran can be transferred safely to a VA or other federal facility, and the VA or other federal facility agrees to accept such a transfer.

[b] Prior to the passage of the Veterans' Emergency Care Fairness Act (P.L. 111-137), a veteran who was enrolled in the VA's health care system was reimbursed for emergency treatment received at a non-VA hospital. However, the statute only permitted such VA reimbursement if the veteran had no other outside health insurance, no matter how limited that other coverage was. P.L. 111-137 would require the VA to pay for emergency treatment for a nonservice-connected condition if a third party is not responsible for paying for the full cost of care. The law also set two limitations on reimbursement as follows: (1) the VA is the secondary payer where a third-party insurer covers a part of the veteran's medical liability (e.g., his or her automobile insurance coverage, private health insurance, or Medicare Part A and Medicare Part B); and (2) the VA is only responsible for the difference between the amount paid by the third-party insurer and the VA allowable amount. Veterans would continue to be responsible for copayments owed to the third-party insurer; if the veteran were responsible for copayments under a private health insurance or Medicare plan, then the veteran would still be liable to pay this (copayment rates and or coinsurance rates are set by the individual insurance policy or Medicare and not the VA). P.L. 111-137 clarifies that veterans are not liable for any remaining balance due to the provider after the third-party insurer and the VA have made their payments.

Does the VA Pay for Medical Care at Non-VA Facilities?

Under certain circumstances, the VA may reimburse non-VA providers for health care services rendered to VA-enrolled veterans on a fee-for-service basis.

Current law authorizes the VA to use Fee Basis Care under the following circumstances: (1) when a clinical service cannot be provided at a VA medical center (VAMC); (2) when a veteran is unable to access VA health care facilities due to geographic inaccessibility; or (3) in emergencies when delays could lead to life-threatening situations.[34] Fee Basis Care may include outpatient care, inpatient care, emergency care, medical transportation, and dental services.[35]

Does the VA Pay for Emergency Care at Non-VA Facilities?

The VA may pay for emergency care provided to enrolled veterans by non-VA providers based on several factors, such as whether the care is for a service-connected condition.

Generally, to be eligible for non-VA emergency care reimbursement veterans must

- be enrolled in the VA health care system, and
- have received VA medical services within the 24-month period preceding the furnishing of emergency treatment.[36]

Once these general eligibility criteria are met, emergency care reimbursement falls into two categories: (1) payment or reimbursement of emergency care for veterans for a service-connected disability[37] and (2) payment or reimbursement of emergency care for veterans for a nonservice-connected disability.[38] The distinct eligibility criteria for each of the two categories are summarized in *Table 2*.

COSTS TO VETERANS AND INSURANCE COLLECTIONS

Do Veterans Have to Pay for Their Care?

Whether a veteran is required to pay for VA health care services depends primarily on (1) whether the condition being treated is service-connected, and/or (2) the veteran's enrollment Priority Group.[39]

Veterans who are enrolled in the VA health care system do not pay any premiums; however, some veterans are required to pay copayments for medical services and outpatient medications related to the treatment of a nonservice-connected condition. *Table 3* summarizes which Priority Groups are charged copayments for inpatient care, outpatient care, outpatient medication, and long-term care services. Only veterans in Priority Group 1 (those who have been rated 50% or more service-connected) and veterans who are deemed catastrophically disabled by a VA provider are never charged a copayment, even for treatment of a nonservice-connected condition. For veterans in other priority groups, VHA currently has four types of nonservice-connected copayments for which veterans may be charged: outpatient, inpatient, extended care services, and medication. Veterans in all priority groups are not charged copayments for a number of outpatient services, including the following: publicly announced VA health fairs; screenings and immunizations; smoking and weight loss counseling; telephone care; laboratory services; flat film radiology; and electrocardiograms.

For primary care outpatient visits, there is a $15 copayment charge and for specialty care outpatient visits, a $50 copayment. Veterans do not receive more than one outpatient copayment charge per day. That is, if the veteran has a primary care visit and a specialty care visit on the same day, the veteran pays only for the specialty care visit. For veterans required to pay an inpatient copayment charge, rates vary based upon whether the veteran is enrolled in Priority Group 7 or not. Veterans enrolled in Priority Group 8 and certain other veterans are responsible for the VA's full inpatient copayment, and veterans enrolled in Priority Group 7 and certain other veterans are responsible for paying 20% of the VA's inpatient copayment. Veterans in Priority Groups 1 through 5 do not have to pay inpatient or outpatient copayments. Veterans in Priority Group 6 may be exempt due to special eligibility for treatment of certain conditions.

For veterans required to pay long-term care copayments, these charges are based on three levels of nonservice-connected care, including inpatient, non-institutional, and adult day health care. Actual copayments vary depending on the veteran's financial situation.

For medication copayments, veterans are not billed if they have a service-connected disability rated 50% or greater, if they are former prisoners of war, or if their medications are related to certain eligibility exceptions. Veterans enrolled in Priority Groups 2 through 6 have a $960 calendar-year cap on the amount that they can be charged for these copayments. Veterans who are unable to pay VA's copayment charges may submit requests for assistance, including waivers, hardships, compromises, and repayment plans.[40]

The VHA bills private health insurers for medical care, supplies, and prescriptions provided to veterans for their nonservice-connected conditions. While the VA cannot bill Medicare, it can bill Medicare supplemental health insurance carriers for covered services.[41] Veterans are not responsible for paying any remaining balance of the VA's insurance claim that is not paid or covered by their health insurance carrier. Any payment received by the VA is used to offset "dollar for dollar" a veteran's VA copayment responsibility.[42]

Can the VA Bill Private Health Insurance?

The VA has the authority to bill most health care insurers for nonservice-connected care provided to veterans enrolled in the VA health care system.

Table 3. Copayments for Health Care Services (CY2012)

	Inpatient care	Outpatient care	Outpatient medication	Long-term care services
	($10/day + $$1,156 for first 90 days and $578 after 90 days; based on 365-day period)	($15 Primary Care; $50 Specialty Care; $0 for x-rays, lab, immunizations, etc.)	($8 per 30-day supply; calendar year cap: $960 for Priority Groups 2-6; $9 for 30-day supply for Priority Groups 7 and 8)[a]	(Institutional nursing home care units, respite care, geriatric evaluation: $0-97 per day. Non-institutional respite care, geriatric evaluation, adult day healthcare: $15 per day; domiciliary care: $5 per day)
Priority Group 1	NO	NO	NO	NO
Priority Group 2[b]	NO	NO	YES	NO
Priority Group 3[b]	NO	NO	YES	NO
Priority Group 4	NO	NO	NO	NO
Priority Group 5[c]	NO	NO	YES	YES
Priority Group 6[d]	NO	NO	NO	NO
Priority Group 7[e]	YES	YES	YES	YES
Priority Group 8[f]	YES	YES	YES	YES

Source: Table prepared by the Congressional Research Service based on information from the Department of Veterans Affairs.

Notes: "NO" means the veteran is not responsible for paying copayments. "YES" means the veteran may be liable for partial or full copayments.

[a] For the period from July 1, 2010, through December 31, 2013, the copayment amount for veterans in Priority Groups 2 through 6 is $8. There is an annual cap of $960 per calendar year. When veterans reach the annual cap, they continue to receive medications without making a copayment. For veterans in Priority Groups 7 and 8 the copayment amount from July 1, 2010, through December 31, 2013, is $9. There is no annual cap for these priority groups.

[b] No medication copayments if medication is for a service-connected disability. Former POWs are exempt from all medication copayments.

[c] No medication or long-term care copayments if veteran is in receipt of VA pension or has an income below applicable pension threshold.

[d] Priority Group 6 are veterans claiming exposure to Agent Orange; veterans claiming exposure to environmental contaminants; veterans exposed to ionizing radiation; combat veterans within five years of discharge from the military; veterans who participated in Project 112/SHAD; veterans claiming military sexual trauma; and veterans with head and neck cancer who received nasopharyngeal radium treatment while in the military are subject to copayments when their treatment or medication is not related to their exposure or experience. The initial registry examination and follow-up visits to receive results of the examination are not billed to the health insurance carrier and are not subject to copayments. However, care provided that is not related to exposure, if it is nonservice-connected, will be billed to the insurance carrier and copayments can apply.

[e] Priority Group 7a and 7c veterans have incomes above the VA Means Test threshold but below the Geographic Means Test threshold and are responsible for 20% of the inpatient copayment and 20% of the inpatient per diem copayment. The Geographic Means Test copayment reduction does not apply to outpatient and medication copayments, and veterans will be assessed the full applicable copayment charges.

[f] Priority Group 8a and 8c veterans have incomes above the VA Means Test threshold and above the Geographic Means Test threshold. Veterans enrolled in these priority groups are responsible for the full inpatient copayment and the inpatient per diem copayment for care of their nonservice-connected conditions. Veterans in these priority groups are also responsible for outpatient and medication copayments for care of their nonserviceconnected conditions.

The Consolidated Omnibus Budget Reconciliation Act of 1985 (P.L. 99-272), enacted into law in 1986, gave the VHA the authority to bill some veterans and most health care insurers for nonservice-connected care provided to veterans enrolled in the VA health care system to help defray the cost of delivering medical services to veterans.[43] This law also established means testing for veterans seeking care for nonservice-connected conditions.

Congress authorized the VHA to collect reasonable charges for medical care or services (including the provision of prescription drugs) from a third party to the extent that the veteran or the provider of the care or services would be eligible to receive payment from the third party for (1) a nonservice-connected disability for which the veteran is entitled to care (or the payment of expenses of care) under a health plan contract;[44] (2) a nonservice-connected disability incurred as a result of the veteran's employment and covered under a worker's compensation law or plan that provides reimbursement or indemnification for such care and services;[45] or (3) a nonserviceconnected disability incurred as a result of a motor vehicle accident in a state that requires automobile accident reparations (no fault) insurance.[46] Similarly, the VHA can receive payments from Medicare supplemental coverage plans for nonservice-connected conditions for which the veterans receives care at VHA facilities.

Veterans are not responsible for paying any remaining balance of the VA's insurance claim not paid or covered by their health insurance. Any payment received by the VA is used to offset "dollar for dollar" a veteran's VA copayment responsibility.[47]

Can the VA Bill Medicare?

The VA is statutorily prohibited from billing Medicare[48] in most situations.

In general, Medicare is prohibited from reimbursing for any services provided by a federal health care provider unless

- the provider is determined by the Secretary of Health and Human Services (HHS) to be providing services to the public as a community institution or agency;
- the provider is providing services through facilities operated by the Indian Health Service (IHS);[49] or
- the services were provided in an emergency (in a hospital setting).

Medicare is also prohibited from making payments to any federal health care provider who is obligated by law or contract to render services at public expense.[50] Therefore, the VHA is statutorily prohibited from receiving Medicare payments for services provided to Medicare-covered veterans.[51] Although the legislative history does not indicate congressional intent for this decision, "a safe assumption to be drawn from the exclusion of Medicare [from paying for health care services provided through other federal entities] is that Congress wanted to avoid the unnecessary transfer of federal funds from Medicare to the VA when the money is all coming out of the same coffer."[52]

It should be noted that there is a narrow exception to this statutory prohibition of Medicare reimbursing the VHA. Under current law the VHA can be reimbursed by Medicare (notwithstanding any condition, limitation, or other provision in title XVIII of the Social Security Act) when the VA provides services to Medicare-covered individuals who are not eligible for care under Chapter 17 of Title 38 United States Code (U.S.C.)[53] and who are afforded VA care or services under a "sharing" agreement.[54]

APPENDIX. VA PRIORITY GROUPS AND THEIR ELIGIBILITY CRITERIA

The VA classifies veterans into eight enrollment Priority Groups based on an array of factors including (but not limited to) service-connected disabilities or exposures,[55] prisoner of war (POW) status, receipt of a Purple Heart or Medal of Honor, and income. The criteria for each Priority Group are summarized in *Table A-1*.

The eight Priority Groups fall into two broad categories. The first group is composed of veterans with service-connected disabilities or with incomes below an established means test. These veterans are regarded by the VA as "high priority" veterans, and they are enrolled in Priority Groups 1-6. Veterans enrolled in Priority Groups 1-6 include the following:

- veterans in need of care for a service-connected disability;
- veterans who have a compensable service-connected condition;
- veterans whose discharge or release from active military, naval, or air service was for a compensable disability that was incurred or aggravated in the line of duty;
- veterans who are former prisoners of war (POWs);
- veterans awarded the Purple Heart;
- veterans who have been determined by the VA to be catastrophically disabled;

Table A-1. VA Priority Groups and Their Eligibility Criteria

Priority Group 1
Veterans with service-connected disabilities rated 50% or more disabling
Veterans determined by VA to be unemployable due to service-connected conditions
Priority Group 2
Veterans with service-connected disabilities rated 30% or 40% disabling
Priority Group 3
Veterans who are former POWsa
Veterans awarded the Purple Heartb
Veterans in receipt of the Medal of Honorc
Veterans whose discharge was for a disability that was incurred or aggravated in the line of duty
Veterans with service-connected disabilities rated 10% or 20% disabling
Veterans awarded special eligibility classification under Title 38, U.S.C., Section 1151, "benefits for individuals disabled
by treatment or vocational rehabilitation"
Priority Group 4
Veterans who are receiving aid and attendance or housebound benefits
Veterans who have been determined by VA to be catastrophically disabled
Priority Group 5
Nonservice-connected veterans and noncompensable service-connected veterans rated 0% disabled whose annual
income and net worth are below the established VA means test thresholds
Veterans receiving VA pension benefits
Veterans eligible for Medicaid benefits
Priority Group 6
Compensable 0% service-connected veterans
Mexican Border War veterans
Veterans solely seeking care for disorders associated with
—exposure to herbicides while serving in Vietnam; or
—ionizing radiation during atmospheric testing or during the occupation of Hiroshima and Nagasaki; or
—service in the Gulf War; or
—being stationed at Camp Lejeune for 30 days or more between January 1, 1957, and December 31, 1987d
—for any illness associated with service in combat in a war after the Gulf War or during a period of hostility after November 11, 1998 as follows:
—Veterans discharged from active duty on or after January 28, 2003, who were enrolled as of January 28, 2008, and veterans who apply for enrollment after January 28, 2008, for five years post discharge
—Veterans discharged from active duty before January 28, 2003, who apply for enrollment after January 28, 2008, until January 27, 2011
Veterans who served on active duty at Camp Lejeune in North Carolina for not less than 30 days during the period beginning on January 1, 1957, and ending on December 31, 1987, for any of the 15 medical conditions specified in 38 U.S.C. 1710(e)(1)(F)e
Priority Group 7

Veterans who agree to pay specified copayments with income and/or net worth above the VA means test threshold and income below the VA national geographic income thresholds
Priority Group 8
Veterans who agree to pay specified copayments with income and/or net worth above the VA means test threshold and the VA national geographic threshold
Subpriority a: Noncompensable 0% service-connected and enrolled as of January 16, 2003, and who have remained enrolled since that date and/or placed in this subpriority due to changed eligibility status
Subpriority b: Noncompensable 0% service-connected and enrolled on or after June 15, 2009, whose income exceeds the current VA means test threshold or VA national geographic income thresholds by 10% or less
Subpriority c: Nonservice-connected veterans enrolled as of January 16, 2003, and who have remained enrolled since that date and/or placed in this subpriority due to changed eligibility status
Subpriority d: Nonservice-connected veterans enrolled on or after June 15, 2009, whose income exceeds the current VA means test threshold or VA national geographic income thresholds by 10% or less
Subpriority e: Noncompensable 0% service-connected veterans not meeting the above criteria Subpriority g: Nonservice-connected veterans not meeting the above criteria

Source: Department of Veterans Affairs.

Notes: Service-connected disability means with respect to disability, that such disability was incurred or aggravated in the line of duty in the active military, naval or air service.

[a] Veterans who are former prisoners of war (POWs) are in Priority Group 3. This began with the enactment of the Former Prisoner of War Benefits Act of 1981 (P.L. 97-37) on August 14, 1981.

[b] Veterans in receipt of a Purple Heart are in Priority Group 3. This began with the enactment of the Veterans Millennium Health Care and Benefits Act (P.L. 106-117) on November 30, 1999.

[c] Veterans in receipt of the Medal of Honor are in Priority Group 3. This began with the enactment of the Caregiver and Veterans Omnibus Health Services Act of 2010 (P.L. 111-163) on May 5, 2010.

[d] The Honoring America's Veterans and Caring for Camp Lejeune Families Act of 2012 (P.L. 112-154), enacted on August 6, 2012, provided this authority.

[e] Veterans who served on active duty at Camp Lejeune in North Carolina between January 1, 1957, and December 31, 1987, are placed in Priority Group 6. These veterans are eligible to receive free medical care for the following 15 illnesses or conditions: esophageal cancer; lung cancer; breast cancer; bladder cancer; kidney cancer; leukemia; multiple myeloma; myleodysplasic syndromes; renal toxicity; hepatic steatosis; female infertility; miscarriage; scleroderma; neurobehavioral effects; and non-Hodgkin's lymphoma. This change occurred with the enactment of the Honoring America's Veterans and Caring for Camp Lejeune Families Act of 2012 (P.L. 112-154) on August 6, 2012.

Table A-2. National Income Thresholds for CY2013

Veterans with—	Free VA prescriptions and travel benefits for veterans with incomes of—	Free VA Heath Care for veterans with incomes of—	Enrollment in Priority Group 8 for veterans with incomes of—
No dependents	$12,465 or less	$30,978 or less	$34,076 or less
1 dependent	$16,324 or less	$37,175 or less	$40,893 or less
2 dependents	$18,453 or less	$39,304 or less	$43,235 or less
3 dependents	$20,582 or less	$41,433 or less	$45,577 or less
4 dependents	$22,711 or less	$43,562 or less	$47,919 or less
For each additional dependent, add:	$2,129	$2,129	$2,129

Source: Department of Veterans Affairs.
Notes: For geographic variations, see http://www.va.gov/healthbenefits/cost/income_thresholds.asp.

- veterans of World War I;
- veterans who were exposed to hazardous agents (such as Agent Orange in Vietnam) while on active duty; and
- veterans who have an annual income and net worth below a VA-established means test threshold.

The VA looks at applicants' income and net worth to determine their specific priority category and whether they have to pay copayments for nonservice-connected care. In addition, veterans are asked to provide the VA with information on any health insurance coverage they have, including coverage through employment or through a spouse. The VA may bill these payers for treatment of conditions that are not a result of injuries or illnesses incurred or aggravated during military service.

The second group of veterans is composed of those who do not fall into one of the first six priority groups—primarily veterans with nonservice-connected medical conditions and with incomes and net worth above the VA-established means test threshold. These veterans are enrolled in Priority Groups 7 or 8.[56]

Table A-2 provides information on income thresholds for VA health care benefits.

End Notes

[1] Department of Veterans Affairs, FY2013 Budget Submission, Medical Programs and Information Technology Programs, Volume 2 of 4, February 2012, p. 1A-3.

[2] U.S. Department of Veterans Affairs, FY 2011 Performance and Accountability Report, Washington, DC, November 15, 2011, p. I-31. Established on January 3, 1946, as the Department of Medicine and Surgery by P.L. 79-293, succeeded in 1989 by the Veterans Health Services and Research Administration, and renamed the Veterans Health Administration in 1991.

[3] Adam Oliver, "The Veterans Health Administration: An American Success Story?" The Milbank Quarterly, vol. 85, no. 1 (March 2007), pp. 5-35.

[4] For a detailed discussion of "promised benefits," see CRS Report 98-1006, Military Health Care: The Issue of "Promised" Benefits, by David F. Burrelli.

[5] Barbara Sydell, "Restructuring the VA Health Care System: Safety Net, Training and Other Considerations," National Health Policy Forum, Issue Brief no. 716, March 1998.

[6] U.S. Congress, House Committee on Veterans Affairs, Veterans' Health Care Eligibility Reform Act of 1996, report to accompany H.R. 3118, 104th Cong. 2nd sess., H.Rept. 104-690, p. 2.

[7] A service-connected disability is a disability that was incurred or aggravated in the line of duty in the U.S. Armed Forces (38 U.S.C. §101 (16)). The VA determines whether veterans have service-connected disabilities, and for those with such disabilities, assigns ratings from 0% to 100% based on the severity of the disability. Percentages are assigned in increments of 10% (38 C.F.R. §§4.1-4.31).

[8] H.Rept. 104-690, p. 5.

[9] Ibid., p. 6.

[10] Ibid., p. 5.

[11] A service-connected disability is a disability that was incurred or aggravated in the line of duty in the U.S. Armed Forces (38 U.S.C. §101 (16)). The VA determines whether veterans have service-connected disabilities, and for those with such disabilities, assigns ratings from 0% to 100% based on the severity of the disability. Percentages are assigned in increments of 10% (38 C.F.R. §§4.1-4.31).

[12] Veterans meeting certain income criteria may be eligible to enroll in the VA without a service-connected condition.

[13] Generally, persons enlisting in one of the Armed Forces after September 7, 1980, and officers commissioned after October 16, 1981, must have completed two years of active duty or the full period of their initial service obligation to be eligible for VA health care benefits. Servicemembers discharged at any time because of service-connected disabilities are not held to this requirement.

[14] A veteran with an "other than honorable" discharge or "bad conduct" discharge may still retain eligibility for VA health care benefits for disabilities incurred or aggravated during service in the military. For more information on the nature of discharge requirements, see CRS Report R42324, "Who is a Veteran?"—Basic Eligibility for Veterans' Benefits, by Christine Scott.

[15] For those servicemembers who are called to duty multiple times, this will be the most recent discharge date. Generally, returning combat veterans are assigned to Priority Group 6, unless eligible for a higher Priority Group, and are not charged copays for medication and/or treatment of conditions that are potentially related to their combat service. At the end of the five-year period, veterans enrolled in Priority Group 6 may be re-enrolled in Priority

Group 7 or 8, depending on their service-connected disability status and income level, and may be required to make copayments for nonservice-connected conditions. The above criteria apply to National Guard and Reserve personnel who were called to active duty by federal executive order and served in a theater of combat operations after November 11, 1998.

[16] A service-connected disability is a disability that was incurred or aggravated in the line of duty in the U.S. Armed Forces (38 U.S.C. §101 (16)). The VA determines whether veterans have service-connected disabilities, and for those with such disabilities, assigns ratings from 0% to 100% based on the severity of the disability. Percentages are assigned in increments of 10% (38 C.F.R. §§4.1-4.31).

[17] A service-connected disability is a disability that was incurred or aggravated in the line of duty in the U.S. Armed Forces (38 U.S.C. §101 (16)). The VA determines whether veterans have service-connected disabilities, and for those with such disabilities, assigns ratings from 0% to 100% based on the severity of the disability. Percentages are assigned in increments of 10% (38 C.F.R. §§4.1-4.31).

[18] 38.U.S.C. §101(24); 38 C.F.R. §3.6(c).

[19] VA Form 10-10EZ is available at https://www.1010ez.med.va.gov/sec/vha/1010ez/. Veterans do not need to apply for enrollment in the VA's health care system if they fall into one of the following categories: veterans with a service-connected disability rated at 50% or more (percentages of disability are based upon the severity of the disability, and those with a rating of 50% or more are placed in Priority Group 1); veterans for whom less than one year has passed since the veteran was discharged from military service for a disability that the military determined was incurred or aggravated in the line of duty, but the VA has not yet rated; or the veteran is seeking care from the VA only for a service-connected disability (even if the rating is only 10%).

[20] H.Rept. 104-690, p. 4.

[21] For example, veterans who may have been exposed to Agent Orange during the Vietnam War or veterans who may have diseases potentially related to service in the Gulf War may be eligible to receive care.

[22] 38 C.F.R. §17.36 (d)(3)(iv) (2009).

[23] For more information on the VA family caregiver program, see http://www.caregiver.va.gov/support_benefits.asp.

[24] Hearing aids and eyeglasses are part of the standard medical package for veterans meeting either of the following criteria: (1) any veteran with a service-connected condition rated 50% or more on one or more disabilities or based on Individual Unemployability or (2) veterans needing care for a service-connected condition.

[25] A detailed listing of the VHA's standard medical benefits package is available at 38 C.F.R. §17.38.

[26] 38 C.F.R. §17.38.

[27] 38 C.F.R. §17.38; and Department of Veterans Affairs, Veterans Health Administration, Health Care Services for Women Veterans, VHA Handbook 1330.01, May 21, 2010.

[28] Department of Veterans Affairs, "VA Dental Insurance Program," 77 Federal Register 12517, March 1, 2012.

[29] 38 C.F.R. §17.149, and Department of Veterans Affairs, Prescribing Hearing Aids and Eyeglasses, VHA Directive 2008-070, October 28, 2008.

[30] Activities of Daily Living (ADLs) generally refer to activities such as bathing, getting in and out of a bed or chair, eating, dressing, walking across the room, and using the toilet.

[31] This section is based on Carol J. Sheets and Heather Mahoney-Gleason, "Caregiver Support in the Veterans Health Administration: Caring For Those Who Care," GENERATIONS – Journal of the American Society on Aging, vol. 34, no. 2 (Summer 2010), pp. 92-98.; U.S. Department of Veterans Affairs, Office of Care Coordination, Supporting Veterans' Caregivers: A Frequently Asked Questions Guide, November 29, 2006, pp. 15-18.; and U.S. Congress, House Committee on Veterans' Affairs, Subcommittee on Health, Legislative Hearing on H.R. 1293, H.R. 1197, H.R. 1302, H.R. 1335, H.R. 1546, H.R. 2734, H.R. 2738, H.R. 2770, H.R. 2898 and Draft Discussion Legislation, 111th Cong., 1st sess., June 18, 2009 (Washington: GPO, 2009), pp. 57-58.

[32] Activities of Daily Living (ADLs) generally refer to activities such as bathing, getting in and out of a bed or chair, eating, dressing, walking across the room, and using the toilet. Instrumental Activities of Daily Living (IADLs) may include activities such as shopping for groceries, light housework, preparing hot meals, using the telephone, taking medications, and managing money.

[33] The CRC program is authorized under 38 U.S.C. §1730.

[34] 38 U.S.C. §§1703, 1725, and 1728.

[35] Department of Veterans Affairs, Veterans Health Administration, Audit of Non-VA Inpatient Fee Care Program, Report No: 09-03408-227, Washington, DC, August 18, 2010, p. 1.

[36] Under current law, "emergency treatment" is defined as medical services furnished, in the judgment of the VA Secretary (1) when VA or other federal facilities are not feasibly available and an attempt to use them beforehand would not be reasonable; (2) when such services are rendered in a medical emergency of such nature that a prudent layperson reasonably expects that delay in seeking immediate medical attention would be hazardous to life or health; and (3) until such time as the veteran can be transferred safely to a VA facility (38 U.S.C. §1725(f)(1)).

[37] 38 U.S.C. §1728.

[38] 38 U.S.C. §1725.

[39] The VA classifies veterans into eight enrollment Priority Groups based on an array of factors including (but not limited to) service-connected disabilities or exposures, prisoner of war (POW) status, receipt of a Purple Heart or Medal of Honor, and income. The criteria for each Priority Group are summarized in the Appendix.

[40] U.S. Congress, House Committee on Veterans' Affairs, Subcommittee on Health, Identifying the Causes of Inappropriate Billing Practices by the U.S. Department of Veterans Affairs, 111th Cong., 1st sess., October 15, 2009 (Washington: GPO, 2010), p. 43.

[41] 38 U.S.C. §1729.

[42] U.S. Congress, House Committee on Veterans' Affairs, Subcommittee on Health, Identifying the Causes of Inappropriate Billing Practices by the U.S. Department of Veterans Affairs, 111th Cong., 1st sess., October 15, 2009 (Washington: GPO, 2010), p. 43.

[43] Veterans' Health-Care and Compensation Rate Amendments of 1985 (P.L. 99-272).

[44] 38 U.S.C. §1729(a)(2)(D), and 38 C.F.R. §17.101(a)(1)(i).

[45] 38 U.S.C. §1729(a)(2)(A), and 38 C.F.R. §17.101(a)(1)(ii).

[46] 38 U.S.C. §1729(a)(2)(B), and 38 C.F.R. §17.101(a)(1)(III).

[47] U.S. Congress, House Committee on Veterans' Affairs, Subcommittee on Health, Identifying the Causes of Inappropriate Billing Practices by the U.S. Department of Veterans Affairs, 111th Cong., 1st sess., October 15, 2009 (Washington: GPO, 2010), p. 43.

[48] "Medicare is a federal insurance program that pays for covered health care services of qualified beneficiaries." CRS Report R40425, Medicare Primer, coordinated by Patricia A. Davis and Scott R. Talaga.

[49] In 1976, Congress authorized Medicare and Medicaid payments for services delivered in Indian health facilities (whether operated by the IHS or Tribes) through amendments to the Social Security Act made in the Indian Health Care Improvement Act of 1976 (P.L. 94-437) (IHCIA). This was permanently authorized by the Patient Protection and Affordable Care Act (PPACA; P.L. 111-148). According to the Centers for Medicare and Medicaid Services American Indian and Alaska Native Strategic Plan 2010–2015: "this entitlement funding was expected to provide critical resources to improve the quality of health care for American Indians and Alaska Natives and to reduce the health status disparities. There is a provision in the IHCIA that Medicaid and Medicare revenues shall not offset congressional appropriations for the IHS, so that the total amount of funding for Indian health care would increase and not merely be shifted from one funding stream to another"(available at http://www.cmsttag.org/docs/CMS%20Strategic%20Plan%20-%20June%2010,%202009%20FINAL.pdf).

[50] 42 U.S.C. §§1395f(c), 1395n(d), 1395f(a).

[51] 42 U.S.C §1395f(c), and 38 U.S.C. §1729(i)(1)(B)(i).

[52] United States v. Blue Cross & Blue Shield of Maryland, Inc., 989 F.2d 718, 727 n. 5 (4th Cir.).

[53] Chapter 17 of Title 38 U.S.C. details the eligibility criteria as well as programs relating to the provision of medical care, and nursing home care, among other things, for veterans and their eligible dependents.

[54] 38 U.S.C. §8153(d). A sharing agreement is a written contract that allows VHA to buy, sell, or exchange health care resources and services with non-VA facilities. VHA could enter into noncompetitive sharing agreements with affiliated institutions (such as affiliated medical schools) and other entities associated with these affiliated institutions (such as university hospitals).

[55] For example, veterans who may have been exposed to Agent Orange during the Vietnam War or veterans who may have diseases potentially related to service in the Gulf War may be eligible to receive care.

[56] The VA considers a veteran's previous year's total household income (both earned and unearned income, as well as his/her spouse's and dependent children's income). Earned income is usually wages received from working. Unearned income includes interest earned, dividends received, money from retirement funds, Social Security payments, annuities, and earnings from other assets. The number of persons in the veterans' family will be factored into the calculation to determine the applicable income threshold. 38 C.F.R. §17.36(b)(7) (2009).

INDEX

A

abuse, 19
access, 14, 20, 26, 27, 28, 37, 43, 51
accounting, 9
adjustment, 11
administrative support, 9
Afghanistan, 42
age, 8, 12, 13, 14, 23, 24, 26, 27
agencies, 8, 21, 47
Alaska, 6, 64
Alaska Natives, 64
amyotrophic lateral sclerosis, 29
APC(s), 25
appointments, 11
appropriations, 7, 21, 29, 38, 64
Appropriations Act, 30
assets, 9, 64
authorities, 4, 7
authority, ix, 9, 12, 13, 25, 36, 38, 54, 55, 59
autism, 29

B

base, 6
beneficiaries, vii, viii, 1, 2, 5, 8, 9, 10, 11, 13, 14, 15, 16, 17, 18, 19, 21, 22, 24, 27, 28, 47, 63
benefits, viii, 12, 13, 14, 18, 19, 21, 24, 26, 27, 36, 40, 42, 43, 58, 60, 61, 62
bladder cancer, 59
bowel, 49
brain, 48
breast cancer, 29, 59

C

cancer, 29, 59
cardiac surgery, 46
caregivers, viii, 35
cataract, 48
category a, 60
certificate, 46
certification, 44
CFR, 25
challenges, 3
children, 10, 11, 13, 24, 64
chronic illness, 47
chronic myelogenous, 29
civil servants, 21
Civilian Health and Medical Program, vii, viii, 2, 9, 36, 41, 47
classes, 16, 44
classification, 58
clinical assessment, 17
clinical judgment, 49
clinical trials, 43
Coast Guard, 9

coding, 25
cognitive impairment, 48
community, 48, 50, 56
compensation, 40, 44, 47, 56
compliance, 6
Congress, 1, 3, 7, 9, 23, 24, 26, 27, 28, 29, 32, 33, 35, 38, 41, 56, 57, 61, 63, 64
Congressional Budget Office, 3, 21, 22, 23, 32, 33
construction, 6, 7, 8, 48
contingency, 14, 28
coordination, 3, 16
cost, 7, 9, 11, 12, 13, 14, 16, 17, 19, 21, 22, 23, 24, 44, 48, 50, 51, 55, 60
cost effectiveness, 16
counseling, ix, 36, 42, 43, 44, 53
covering, 6, 17

D

daily living, 46, 48, 49
deficiencies, 48
dental care, ix, 20, 36, 44, 46
dental plans, viii, 2, 10
Department of Defense, vii, 1, 7, 8, 10, 29, 31, 32, 33
deposits, 8
diabetes, 47
directives, 4
directors, 4
disabilities, viii, 19, 35, 37, 61, 62
disability, 13, 14, 19, 24, 38, 39, 44, 45, 47, 50, 52, 53, 55, 56, 57, 58, 59, 61, 62
diseases, 29, 47, 62, 64
District of Columbia, 6, 19
doctors, 7
drugs, 16, 17, 18, 43, 47

E

earnings, 64
education, 5, 31, 49
eligibility criteria, 44, 51, 52, 64
emergency, ix, 36, 50, 51, 52, 56, 63

employees, viii, 35, 36
employment, 46, 47, 56, 60
endangered, 31
end-stage renal disease, 13, 24
enrollment, 11, 13, 14, 19, 24, 27, 37, 38, 39, 40, 41, 52, 57, 58, 62, 63
equipment, ix, 18, 36, 43
esophageal cancer, 59
ESRD, 13, 14
exclusion, 57
execution, 4
expenditures, 26
exposure, 55, 58

F

families, 11, 12, 14, 15
family members, 11, 12, 14, 15, 19, 20, 41
FDA, 43
federal facilities, 50, 63
federal funds, 57
federal government, 37
Federal Register, 25, 32, 62
fertilization, ix, 36, 43, 44
fetus, 31
financial, 40, 41, 53
Food and Drug Administration, 17, 43
force, 22, 24
formula, 26
funding, 6, 7, 8, 29, 31, 64
funds, viii, 2, 64

G

GAO, 3
generic drugs, 17, 18
Georgia, 6
glasses, 47
governor, 40
grades, 11, 17, 19
grants, 29
growth, 18, 21, 22
growth rate, 21
guidance, 4, 29

Index

H

Hawaii, 5, 6
hazards, 37
head and neck cancer, 55
health, vii, viii, ix, 1, 2, 3, 5, 6, 7, 8, 9, 10, 12, 16, 19, 20, 21, 22, 23, 24, 25, 26, 28, 29, 31, 32, 35, 36, 37, 38, 39, 40, 41, 43, 44, 49, 50, 51, 52, 53, 54, 55, 56, 60, 61, 62, 63, 64
Health and Human Services, 24, 56
health care, vii, viii, ix, 1, 2, 6, 7, 8, 11, 16, 20, 21, 22, 23, 24, 25, 26, 28, 35, 36, 37, 38, 39, 40, 41, 43, 44, 49, 51, 52, 53, 54, 55, 56, 60, 61, 62, 63, 64
health care costs, viii, 2, 22, 23, 24
health care system, 21, 37, 41, 51, 52, 54, 55, 62
health information, 5
health insurance, 9, 22, 26, 41, 50, 51, 53, 55, 56, 60
health services, 19, 43
health status, 64
hearing impairment, 48
heart attack, 39, 40
HHS, 24, 56
history, 56
home care services, 49
homes, 49, 50
hospice, 43
host, 48
hostilities, 5
hostility, 58
House, 30, 33, 61, 63
House of Representatives, 33
household income, 64
housing, 49
human, 4
human resources, 4

I

in vitro, ix, 36, 43, 44

income, viii, 26, 35, 37, 38, 39, 40, 41, 55, 57, 58, 60, 61, 62, 63, 64
independence, 46
Indians, 64
individuals, 12, 13, 14, 24, 57, 58
infection, 46
infertility, ix, 36, 43, 59
inflation, 21, 22
injuries, 49, 60
injury, 39, 40, 47, 50
institutions, 64
insurance policy, 51
investment, 9
ionizing radiation, 55, 58
Iowa, 6
Iraq, 42
issues, viii, 2, 3, 4

K

kidney, 59

L

laws, 28
layperson, 63
lead, 51
leadership, 3
legislation, 17
leukemia, 29, 59
lifetime, 28
light, 63
logistics, 5
Louisiana, 6
lung cancer, 59
lymphoma, 59

M

management, 9, 45, 46
manpower, 3, 4
manufacturing, 18
Marine Corps, 3
Maryland, 6, 64

matter, 51
Medicaid, 24, 37, 41, 58, 64
medical, vii, viii, ix, 1, 4, 5, 6, 7, 8, 13, 14, 17, 18, 20, 21, 23, 24, 26, 27, 28, 29, 31, 35, 36, 37, 38, 40, 41, 42, 43, 44, 45, 46, 47, 48, 49, 50, 51, 52, 53, 55, 56, 58, 59, 60, 62, 63, 64
medical care, viii, ix, 5, 14, 21, 23, 24, 26, 27, 28, 35, 36, 41, 44, 49, 53, 56, 59, 64
medical history, 26
Medicare, vii, viii, ix, 2, 7, 8, 9, 13, 24, 25, 26, 27, 31, 32, 33, 36, 37, 41, 50, 51, 53, 56, 57, 63, 64
medication, ix, 17, 18, 36, 44, 52, 53, 54, 55, 61
medicine, viii, 2, 17
membership, 43
mental health, 42, 43
mental retardation, 19
Mexico, 6
military, vii, viii, ix, 1, 2, 3, 4, 5, 7, 8, 11, 13, 14, 15, 16, 20, 21, 23, 24, 26, 27, 28, 29, 35, 36, 37, 38, 39, 40, 44, 46, 55, 57, 59, 60, 61, 62
military health system, vii, viii, 1, 2, 3, 5, 7, 21
miscarriage, 59
mission(s), vii, 1, 5, 9, 21
Missouri, 6
MOG, 4
Montana, 6
multiple myeloma, 59
multiple sclerosis, 47

N

National Defense Authorization Act, 8, 12, 13, 18, 23, 24, 25, 27, 31, 32, 33, 39
nursing, ix, 19, 36, 48, 49, 54, 64
nursing care, ix, 36, 48, 49
nursing home, 48, 49, 54, 64

O

Obama, 7, 41
Obama Administration, 7
occupational therapy, 49
Oklahoma, 6
operations, 4, 6, 27, 38, 39, 62
oral health, 44, 45
organ, 46
outpatient, viii, ix, 14, 21, 22, 25, 36, 41, 42, 43, 51, 52, 53, 55
ovarian cancer, 29
oversight, 4, 5, 9

P

palliative, 43
participants, 11, 12
pathology, 49
PCM, 15
penalties, 27
permit, 26
Persian Gulf, 38
Persian Gulf War, 38
pharmaceutical(s), ix, 16, 17, 18, 21, 36
pharmacy, viii, 2, 5, 16, 17, 18, 21, 23, 24
Philadelphia, 16
photosensitivity, 47
physical therapy, 49
policy, 4, 5, 20, 31
population, 25
POWER, 4
pregnancy, 31, 33
prescription drugs, 15, 18, 21, 42, 43, 56
President, 7, 9, 10, 23, 24, 41
Priority Groups, viii, 35, 37, 41, 52, 53, 54, 55, 57, 58, 60, 63
prisoners, 37, 47, 53, 57, 59
prisoners of war, 37, 47, 53, 57, 59
private sector, 21
prosthetic device, ix, 36
psychological health, 29
public health, 5
Puerto Rico, 19

Index

R

radium, 55
rape, 31, 33
RE, 32
real property, 6
recognition, 13
recommendations, 16, 22, 23
reconstruction, 5
recruiting, 28
reform, 26, 31, 37, 41, 61
regulations, ix, 28, 36, 44
rehabilitation, 45, 46
rehabilitation program, 45, 46
reimburse, ix, 7, 36, 50, 51
requirements, viii, 5, 16, 18, 25, 35, 38, 44, 48, 61
research funding, 29
Residential, 49
resource management, 4, 5
resources, 4, 6, 7, 37, 38, 50, 64
restrictions, 27
retail, 15, 16, 17, 18, 21
retirement, 11, 12, 18, 64
rodents, 31
rules, 25, 30

S

school, 64
scleroderma, 59
sclerosis, 29
scope, 44
Secretary of Defense, 3, 5, 8, 9, 13, 18, 24, 28, 32
Senate, 30
service-connected disabilities, viii, ix, 35, 36, 37, 41, 45, 57, 58, 61, 62, 63
services, vii, ix, 1, 5, 6, 7, 9, 10, 13, 17, 18, 19, 20, 21, 25, 26, 27, 36, 37, 38, 39, 41, 43, 44, 46, 47, 48, 49, 51, 52, 53, 54, 55, 56, 57, 63, 64
sex, 10
smoking, 53

Social Security, 24, 26, 33, 57, 64
social services, 49
South Dakota, 6
special education, 18
specialists, 11
speech, 49
spending, 26
spinal cord, 49
stabilization, 50
state(s), 20, 38, 40, 48, 56
stock, 16
stroke, 39, 40, 47
structure, 27
subsidy, 12
substance abuse, 43
supervision, 49, 50
support services, 49
survivors, viii, 19, 20, 35, 41, 47

T

target, 26
Task Force, 5, 22, 23, 32
taxes, 26
technology, 5
teeth, 45
telephone, 53, 63
testing, ix, 36, 47, 55, 58
tooth, 45
toxic substances, 37
toxicity, 47, 59
training, 5, 27, 31, 39, 42, 45
transplant, 46
transportation, ix, 36, 51
trauma, ix, 31, 36, 44, 45, 55
traumatic brain injury, 29, 47
treatment, vii, ix, 1, 5, 6, 13, 14, 15, 16, 36, 44, 45, 46, 47, 48, 49, 50, 51, 52, 53, 55, 58, 60, 61, 63
treatment facilities, vii, 1, 5, 6, 13, 15, 16
TRICARE Extra, vii, 2, 9, 11, 13, 14

U

United States, 7, 19, 28, 57, 64

V

valuation, 32
variations, 60
victims, 19
Vietnam, 58, 60, 62, 64
vision, ix, 36, 47, 48
vocational rehabilitation, 45, 46, 58

W

wages, 64
walking, 62, 63
war, 7, 39, 41, 45, 57, 58, 63
Washington, 4, 6, 61, 63
web, 15, 32
weight loss, 53
Wisconsin, 6
World War I, 37, 60
worldwide, vii, 1, 5, 12

X

x-rays, 44, 54